PRINCIPLES OF MEDICINE AND MEDICAL NURSING

MODERN NURSING SERIES

General Editors:
SUSAN E. NORMAN, SRN, NDN Cert, RNT
Senior Tutor, The Nightingale School, St. Thomas's Hospital, London

JEAN HEATH, BA, SRN, SCM, Cert Ed
National Health Learning Resources Unit, Sheffield City Polytechnic

Consultant Editor:
A J HARDING RAINS, MS, FRCS
Regional Dean, British Postgraduate Medical Federation;
formerly Professor of Surgery, Charing Cross Hospital Medical School,
University of London; Honorary Consultant Surgeon, Charing Cross Hospital;
Honorary Consultant Surgeon to the Army

This series caters for the needs of a wide range of nursing, medical and ancillary professions. Some of the titles are given below, but a complete list is available from the Publisher.

Community Health and Social Services
J B MEREDITH DAVIES, MD, FFCM, DPH

Nursing – Image or Reality?
MARGARET C SCHURR, SRN, NACert, Cert Ed. and JANET TURNER, SRN, SCM, Dip N

Communicable Diseases
WILFRID H PARRY, MD, DPH, DTM and H

Gerontology and Geriatric Nursing
SIR W FERGUSON ANDERSON, OBE, KStJ, MD, FRCP
F I CAIRD, MA, DM, FRCP, R D KENNEDY, MB ChB, FRCP and
DORIS SCHWARTZ, MA, RN

Obstetrics and Gynaecology
JOAN M E QUIXLEY, SRN, RNT and MICHAEL D CAMERON, MA, MB, BChir, FRCS, ARCOG

Taverner's Physiology
DERYCK TAVERNER, MBE, MD, FRCP

General Surgery and the Nurse
R E HORTON, MBE, MS, FRCS (Eng)

Intensive Care
A K YATES, MB, ChB, FRCS, P J MOORHEAD, MB, ChB, MRCP and A P ADAMS, PhD, MD, BS, FFARCS

Community Child Health
MARION E JEPSON, MBE, MB, ChB, DCH, DPH, FFCM

PRINCIPLES OF MEDICINE AND MEDICAL NURSING

Sixth Edition

J C Houston
CBE, MD, FRCP
Dean of the United Medical and Dental
Schools of Guy's and St. Thomas's Hospitals

Hilary Hyde White
SRN, RNT
Senior Nurse Tutor, Post-Basic and
Continuing Education, East Roding School of Nursing

HODDER AND STOUGHTON
LONDON SYDNEY AUCKLAND TORONTO

British Library Cataloguing in Publication Data

Houston, J. C.
Principles of medicine and medical nursing.
—6th ed.—(Modern nursing series)
1. Pathology 2. Nursing
I. Title II. White, Hilary Hyde III. Series
616'.0024613 RT65

ISBN 0 340 34450 4

First published 1958 Reprinted 1962, 1963, 1965
Second edition 1966 Reprinted 1968, 1969
Third edition 1972 Reprinted 1974
Fourth edition 1975 Reprinted 1977
Fifth edition 1979 Reprinted 1980, 1982
Sixth edition 1985
This book was first published under the authorship of J. C. Houston and Marion G. Stockdale. The third and subsequent editions were revised by J. C. Houston and Hilary Hyde White

Printed in Great Britain for
Hodder and Stoughton Educational,
a division of Hodder and Stoughton Ltd.,
Mill Road, Dunton Green, Sevenoaks, Kent
by Richard Clay (The Chaucer Press) Ltd,
Bungay, Suffolk

Photo Typeset by Macmillan India Ltd., Bangalore.

Editors' Foreword

This well established series of books reflects contemporary nursing and health care practice. It is used by a wide range of nursing, medical and ancillary professions and encompasses titles suitable for different levels of experience from those in training to those who have qualified.

Members of the nursing professions need to be highly informed and to keep critically abreast of demanding changes in attitudes and technology. The series therefore continues to grow with new titles being added to the list and existing titles being updated regularly. Its aim is to promote sound understanding by presenting essential facts clearly and concisely. We hope this will lead to nursing care of the highest standard.

Preface

In the sixth edition of this popular textbook many amendments and additions have been made throughout the text and in particular new sections on Legionnaire's disease, spontaneous pneumothorax, respiratory failure, intensive care and bereavement, genital herpes and toxocariasis have been incorporated. The elimination of smallpox from the world has made it possible for this section to be deleted and in view of the virtual elimination of poliomyelitis from the UK this section has been vigorously pruned. We believe this new section provides a lucid and balanced account of the common medical problems encountered by nurses today.

It remains the principal object of the book to give the nurse a clear appreciation of how the symptoms and signs of disease arise, in a simple but accurate form. With this knowledge she can best perform the vital service of reassuring the worried patient by helping him to understand his own condition and, of particular importance to those with chronic disorders, encouraging him to learn to live with his disabilities.

We should like to thank those from Guy's who, in their various capacities, helped with the book at its inception. In particular we should like to thank the Dietetic Department for allowing us to use their scheme for a high fibre diet. Above all we are grateful to Marion Stockdale, formerly Principle Sister Tutor at Guy's, who as one of the original authors of the book contributed so much on which subsequent editions have built.

Contents

Editors' Foreword v
Preface vi

1 The Cardiovascular System 1
2 Disorders of the Blood and Lymphatic System 30
3 The Respiratory System 42
4 Intensive Care Nursing 75
5 The Alimentary System 78
6 The Urinary System 105
7 Vitamins 113
8 The Endocrine System 117
9 The Chronic Rheumatic Diseases and the Collagen Diseases 131
10 The Nervous System 139
11 Diseases of the Skin 173
12 Infectious Diseases 184
13 Caring for Mentally Ill Patients 210
14 Venereal Diseases 214
15 Diseases Due to Worms (HELMINTHS) 221

Glossary 224
Diets 227
Approximate Equivalent Doses 233
Conversion Scales for SI Units 235
Index 237

I

The Cardiovascular System

A. Examination of the Cardiac Patient

1. *General Examination*

Cyanosis The colour of a part in terms of its redness or its pallor depends on the amount of blood in the small vessels (capillaries) of the part—where the overlying tissue is thin, e.g. lips and conjunctiva, the colour may be very marked. As it is haemoglobin which gives the blood its colour, the amount of haemoglobin in blood will influence the intensity, and the condition of the haemoglobin will influence the shade of colour produced. When the haemoglobin is well oxygenated the tissues will look pink, and as the haemoglobin gives up its oxygen the tissues will begin to acquire a bluish tinge. When blood contains as much as 5 g per cent of reduced haemoglobin, tissues containing such blood look blue and the condition is known as 'cyanosis'. Now, patients with severe anaemia may have less than 5 g of haemoglobin per 100 ml of blood, and therefore they can never show cyanosis; on the other hand, in the condition known as polycythaemia, in which there is a great excess of red blood corpuscles, the blood contains so much haemoglobin that more than 5 g per 100 ml is always in the de-oxygenated state, and the patients are therefore always cyanosed. Healthy people often show some degree of cyanosis in cold weather; this is because the blood circulates more slowly through the capillaries of the exposed parts and the tissues are able to remove more oxygen from it. Similarly, cyanosis occurs in cardiac failure partly from the slowing of the circulation, but partly because pulmonary congestion prevents adequate oxygenation of the blood passing through the lungs. In some forms of congenital heart disease (blue babies) deep cyanosis is seen because a proportion of the venous blood in the right side of the heart takes a short cut into the aorta and does not pass through the lungs at all.

The temperature of a part depends on the blood flow to the part, so that any diminution in flow will tend to produce coldness.

Coldness of the extremities results from the fall in cardiac output and slowing of the circulation which usually occur in heart failure; in patients whose cardiac output remains high, however—

for example, those with thyrotoxic heart failure—the extremities remain warm.

Dyspnoea, orthopnoea and **oedema** are considered on p. 6.

2. *The Pulse*

When taking the pulse it is a good plan to study first the condition of the arterial wall. To do this, two fingers must be used, so that the pulse-wave may be obliterated with the more proximal finger while the more distal one palpates the artery. Otherwise the pressure of the blood in the vessel may give an erroneous impression of the hardness of its wall. In healthy young people the artery can only just be felt when the pulse has been obliterated by pressure higher up, whereas the changes of arteriosclerosis cause it to be not only more rigid, so that it can easily be felt, but also very tortuous in its course.

The pulse-wave should next be considered and the following points noted:

Rate During the first year of life the normal resting pulse-rate is about 100 per minute. As the child grows the pulse becomes slower, and by puberty it has settled down to the adult rate, which usually lies between about 65 and 85 beats per minute. Athletes, however, may have a normal pulse rate of 50 or even less. Increase in the pulse-rate (tachycardia) may be due to emotion, exertion, fever, thyrotoxicosis or heart failure; sleep eliminates the first of these causes, and therefore the sleeping pulse-rate is often a valuable observation. Slowing of the pulse (bradycardia) is less common; it may be due to heart-block, over-dosage with digitalis, hypothyroidism or raised intracranial pressure.

Rhythm

Anatomy and Physiology The beating of the heart is controlled by a regular series of electrical impulses discharged at intervals of usually slightly under a second from the sino-atrial node. The impulse spreads first to the two atria and causes them to contract. It then reaches the atrio-ventricular node, and travels from there down the atrio-ventricular bundle, which delivers it simultaneously to the two ventricles and causes them to contract. Normally it takes the impulse about a fifth of a second to pass down the bundle from the atria to the ventricles, and this interval allows the atria time to empty their blood into the ventricles before they in turn contract and eject it into the aorta and pulmonary artery. When the atrio-ventricular bundle is unable to transmit some or all of the atrial impulses to the ventricles, the patient is said to have partial or complete heart-block. Although the normal pulse is usually regular in time and force, there are two types of irregularity which are commonly found in healthy people:

(1) **Sinus Arrhythmia** is a condition characterised by rhythmical fluctuation of the rate of discharge from the sino-atrial node and is detected by asking the patient to take a deep breath, since in this condition the heart-rate becomes faster during inspiration and slower during expiration. It is usually found in young people, and is a positive sign of cardiac health.

(2) **Extra Systoles** are not in fact extra beats, but premature ones arising not from the normal sino-atrial node but from another point somewhere in the muscle of the atria or ventricles. As the beat comes prematurely, the ventricle is only partially filled, so that the beat is smaller than normal; and as the refractory period which follows it prevents the development of the next normal impulse, there is then a compensatory pause, during which more blood flows into the ventricle than normal, so that the next beat is unusually forceful. Occasional extra systoles are quite common in healthy people and are sometimes related to over-indulgence in tobacco or alcohol; they are also often found, however, in patients with heart disease, so that their significance in a particular patient can be decided only after assessing the rest of the clinical evidence. The patient frequently fails to detect the extra systole, but notes the compensatory pause to which he refers as 'a dropped beat'.

The more serious causes of arrhythmia are:

(1) **Atrial Fibrillation.** In this condition the regular co-ordinated contraction of the atria initiated by impulses from the sino-atrial node is replaced by frequent fibrillary twitches in isolated muscle bundles in the atrial walls, which send some 300 irregularly spaced impulses per minute down the atrio-ventricular bundle. As the bundle usually cannot transmit at this speed, the consequent partial heart-block reduces the ventricular rate from the potential 300 to perhaps about 150 irregular beats per minute. Some of these beats occur when there is so little blood in the ventricle that no pulse-wave is transmitted to the peripheral arteries. Subtraction of the pulse-rate from the apex beat-rate therefore gives the **pulse deficit**,

which is a measure of the number of ineffective beats the heart is making each minute. The pulse is completely irregular in time and force. Atrial fibrillation occurs particularly in patients with rheumatic heart disease, coronary artery disease or thyrotoxic heart disease. Less often it results from severe infection or toxaemia, and occasionally paroxysms of fibrillation occur in apparently healthy people.

(2) **Atrial Flutter** is very similar in its causation and effects to fibrillation, but the rapid beats are regular in timing.

(3) **Paroxysmal Tachycardia** results from the regular discharge of a rapid series of impulses from an abnormal focus in the atria or ventricles. Heart-block (see p. 3) usually reduces the ventricular rate to half or a third of the atrial rate, and as the block often varies quite suddenly in degree, the rate at the wrist may be doubled or halved while the pulse is being taken.

(4) **Pulsus Bigeminus,** or coupling of the heart, occurs when a premature systole and compensatory pause follow each normal beat. Typically the pulse reveals a succession of double beats, each pair being separated by a pause; sometimes, however, the second beat of each pair is so weak that it cannot be felt, and the condition can then be detected only by auscultation of the heart. The commonest cause of coupled beats is over-dosage with digitalis.

(5) **Pulsus Alternans** is the condition in which alternate strong and weak beats occur at approximately regular intervals. When the difference in the strength of the alternate beats is only slight it cannot be detected by feeling the pulse, but it is quite easy to demonstrate it when the blood pressure is taken. Pulsus alternans is in fact usually found in patients with high blood pressure; it is a sign of weakness in the myocardium of the left ventricle and therefore usually implies a poor prognosis.

B. Heart Failure

It is important to understand what is meant by the term heart failure and to distinguish it clearly from the various types of heart disease. To this end a brief résumé of the normal functions of the heart will be helpful. Venous blood returning to the heart from all parts of the body is delivered via the superior and inferior venae cavae into the right atrium and then flows through the tricuspid valve into the right ventricle. Contraction of the right ventricle pumps it into the blood vessels of the lungs, where it gives off carbon dioxide and takes up oxygen. The oxygenated blood returns along the pulmonary veins to the left atrium and thence through the mitral valve into the left ventricle, which ejects it into the aorta, from where it is distributed all over the body. The work of the heart therefore falls mainly on the two ventricles. In healthy people these are powerful muscular chambers with ample reserves of strength: that is to say, when as a result of strenuous exertion there is a demand by the muscles and other tissues for more oxygen and other nutriments, the ventricles can pump on many times more blood than under resting conditions and still show no symptoms of strain or failure.

The various diseases which affect the heart make inroads, sometimes gradually and sometimes suddenly, into the strength which the ventricles hold in reserve. The consequence is that when, say, half this functional reserve has been destroyed the patient finds he can do only half as much extra work before symptoms of distress appear; and therefore in following the progress of his disease the most helpful method is to see how much physical work he can do, for example, how many steps he can climb before he has to rest.

The symptoms and signs of heart failure are due partly to the deficiency of arterial blood being delivered to the tissues, but more conspicuously to the accumulation of blood which occurs upstream to the failing chamber, or chambers, of the heart. Although in most cases there is eventually failure of the whole heart, there is often at first evidence of failure affecting only the ventricle which has borne the main burden of the disease; it is therefore helpful to consider separately left ventricular failure and right ventricular failure.

Left Ventricular Failure

The left ventricle has more work to do

(1) when there is a raised blood pressure in the systemic arteries, since it has to eject its blood into the aorta against an increased resistance;

(2) when there is stenosis (narrowing) of the aortic valve, so that again blood has to be forced with greater difficulty into the aorta, and

(3) when there is aortic regurgitation, so that the ventricle has to pump out not only the normal amount of blood which has reached it in the usual way but also the amount which has leaked back into it during the preceding diastole. At first the ventricle responds to this increased load by undergoing what is called 'work hypertrophy': the muscle-fibres within its wall increase in size and strength, and this

process enables it for a time to maintain a normal circulation. Eventually, however, the strain tells. The ventricle can no longer pump sufficient blood into the aorta, and the accumulation of blood upstream to the failing chamber causes distension of the left atrium and of the pulmonary veins which drain into it. This congestion of the pulmonary blood vessels makes the lungs more rigid than normal and impedes the movements of respiration, so that the main symptom of left ventricular failure is **dyspnoea** or difficulty in breathing. This may come on gradually, being noticed at first only on exertion, but frequently the pulmonary congestion occurs acutely during the night, the patient waking in a state of great alarm with a sense of suffocation and fighting for his breath. Such an attack is called **cardiac asthma**. It usually subsides in an hour or so with the expectoration of a little frothy sputum. The recumbent position tends to increase pulmonary congestion; that is why the patient with left heart failure gets cardiac asthma during the night and eventually finds he has to remain more or less upright in order to breathe comfortably. The state of breathlessness which necessitates this upright position is known as **orthopnoea.**

Acute L.V. failure is often due to myocardial infarction (p. 22).

Right Heart Failure

Failure of the right side of the heart is usually seen in patients who already have dyspnoea and orthopnoea from the pulmonary congestion of left-sided failure. Occasionally, however, it occurs alone, as for example when congenital stenosis of the pulmonary artery or a disease of the lungs such as emphysema puts a strain solely upon the right ventricle. Again failure results in accumulation of blood upstream to the failing chamber. Blood collects first in the right atrium and venae cavae and later all the systemic veins in the body are distended with blood under increased pressure. For the diagnosis of right heart failure we look therefore not at the heart itself but at the veins. The most convenient vein to study is usually the external jugular vein in the neck: in normal people who are sitting upright or reclining at not less than 45° this vein is collapsed and empty, but in right heart failure the increased venous pressure causes it to remain distended with blood in this position. The general increase in venous pressure impedes the re-absorption into the bloodstream of tissue fluid, which therefore accumulates and can be detected as pitting **oedema**. In patients who are up this is found round the feet and ankles; in those confined to bed it forms a pad over the sacrum and lumbar region. For similar reasons in severe congestive heart failure fluid also collects in the peritoneal cavity, where it is called ascites, and in the pleural cavities. Engorgement of the veins of the stomach and intestines often causes some digestive upset, usually with loss of appetite and flatulence; while distension of the liver with blood causes this organ to be enlarged, often painful and nearly always tender. The accumulation of fluid in the tissues inevitably means that less is being eliminated by the kidneys; the urine in heart failure is therefore scanty and highly concentrated and frequently contains a little protein.

In severe failure usually affecting the whole heart the fall in cardiac output of blood causes the patient's extremities to be cold and his pulse weak. Cyanosis is the blue colour which results when the blood contains more de-oxygenated haemoglobin than normal (see p. 1); in cardiac failure the reasons for this are the slowing of the circulation, which gives the tissues time to withdraw more oxygen than normal from the blood, and the congestion of the lungs, which prevents its adequate oxygenation there. Alternate strong and weak beats of the pulse (**pulsus alternans**) usually indicate serious weakness of the left ventricle and imply a grave prognosis. **Cheyne-Stokes** respiration is a particular type of periodic breathing: after a phase in which the breaths come with increasingly rapid speed and amplitude to a climax and then subside again there is a phase of complete cessation of breathing before the cycle starts again. Each phase may last half a minute or so. This type of respiration is seen particularly in elderly people with heart failure, usually in the terminal stages of the illness, and is probably due to the lack of an adequate blood supply to the respiratory centre in the brain.

Treatment and Nursing Care In no other disease is rest more important than in the treatment of heart failure, the aim being to rest the heart, the body and the mind.

The patient is nursed in bed, well supported by pillows, and may find breathing easier if he leans forward resting his arms on a bed-table. This upright position must be maintained particularly when there is left-sided failure with cardiac asthma and pulmonary oedema. If an adjustable bed is available, the patient will be able to sit up with the legs lowered, so diminishing the venous return to the heart and reducing the pulmonary congestion. An excellent alternative is a high-backed arm-chair; many patients find this more comfortable, and so rest and sleep more easily. The patient's position must be changed frequently and the usual treatment for pressure areas given. For an attack of cardiac asthma an intramuscular injection of morphine 15–20 mg, perhaps combined with frusemide 40 mg IV, is very beneficial: fear is allayed, restlessness and dyspnoea subside and sleep often follows, with resulting great general improvement. The administration of oxygen, by Venti-mask, is often indicated for the relief of anoxia. A diuretic must be given to reduce the blood volume and so lower the venous pressure; this relieves the over-filling of the heart, resulting in a rise in cardiac output and reduction in oedema. For rapid effect in acute left ventricular failure 20 mg of frusemide intravenously is very effective. Aminophylline 0.5 g intravenously is also a very useful drug in this condition, particularly in relieving Cheyne-Stokes respiration.

Digitalis is another important drug used in the treatment of heart failure; it is most commonly given in the form of Digoxin. Digitalis is a cumulative drug: a relatively large dose is given for the first few days, therefore, and when a good therapeutic concentration has accumulated in the body the dosage must be reduced, so that thereafter the patient takes in just as much as he excretes, and in this way maintains the correct concentration in his tissues. If the original large dose is continued, the patient will continue to accumulate the digitalis in his body with possibly dangerous results. Initial dosage might be Digoxin 0.25 mg four times daily, reducing the administration to twice or three times daily after a few days: if the patient is very gravely ill, and *providing he has not had any digitalis recently*, a slow intravenous injection of Digoxin 0.5–0.75 mg may be given.

The beneficial effect of digitalis is partly due to its action in reducing the conductivity of the atrio-ventricular bundle, whereby many of the excessive number of stimuli from the atria are prevented from reaching the ventricles. In addition, digitalis directly stimulates the heart-muscle to more powerful contraction. The ventricles therefore beat less frequently and more forcibly, and as the filling time is lengthened, each beat becomes a useful beat. The improvement is revealed, therefore, not only by slowing of the heart but also by reduction in the pulse deficit, and to show this every patient with atrial fibrillation must have both the apex and radial rates taken and recorded every 4 hours. Digitalis being a cumulative drug, watch must be kept for signs of over-dosage, which is suggested by nausea and vomiting, slowing of the pulse to 60 or below, pulsus bigeminus (p. 0) or atrial tachycardia. As a precautionary measure the pulse-rate must be taken immediately before giving every dose. Toxic effects are more common in elderly patients and in those with potassium deficiency (which often results from the use of the thiazide diuretics).

The patient will have no desire for food during the first few days, but nourishing drinks should be given in moderate amounts. When food is given it should be dry and in small quantities at frequent intervals. The nurse can do a great deal to encourage her patient to eat by finding out the foods preferred, by offering those which are easily digested and by serving them attractively. At times it may be necessary to feed the patient, but this often worries him, and if it does he will be less distressed if he is allowed to feed himself. Failure to eliminate enough sodium in the urine is one of the main causes of oedema in heart failure, since sodium has the property of retaining in the tissues an osmotically equivalent volume of water. The salt in the diet therefore has to be restricted. No salt should be added and foods containing high salt levels should be avoided.

Diuretics In chronic heart failure an oral diuretic is given for the relief of oedema. Most patients do well on bendrofluazide 2.5–5 mg on alternate mornings; if a more powerful effect is needed frusemide 40–120 mg may be substituted.

As these drugs cause potassium depletion potassium supplements (such as 'Slow K') must also be given. By contrast, triamterene (200 mg daily) and amiloride (10–40 mg daily) are powerful diuretics which cause potassium retention. The addition of spironolactone 25–100 mg four times daily may help to clear obstinate oedema; it antagonises aldosterone, the salt-retaining hormone of the adrenal cortex. Occasionally some patients fail to respond to diuretics; if the oedema is gross, fluid may have to be removed by pleural and peritoneal aspirations or incisions through the skin of the legs.

A tranquilliser such as diazepam 2–5 mg t.d.s. may be very helpful in promoting rest and freedom from anxiety.

Oxygen This should be administered to anoxic patients; it relieves dyspnoea and by ensuring an adequate blood oxygen level prevents the heart having to beat quickly to oxygenate the tissues. Oxygen should be prescribed by a doctor and only administered according to instructions.

Management At all times the patient must be spared from any unnecessary physical or emotional strain. Often the use of a commode or wheeling the patient in a chair to the toilet is less exhausting for him than using a bedpan. At the same time the bed can be made, and so one more tax on the patient's strength is avoided. Furthermore, this short time out of bed each day helps not only in improving the patient's morale but also in diminishing the tendency to thrombosis in the deep veins of the legs, a complication which is favoured by the sluggish venous circulation in patients with heart failure. Chest infections and deep vein thrombosis in the legs are likely complications which can be averted by exercises from the physiotherapist and nurse. The bed clothes should be light and where necessary kept off the patient by a bed cradle.

By the nature of their illness such patients may be irritable and depressed. The nurse needs great patience, understanding and firm kindness to help them.

To prevent unnecessary relapses and admission to hospital, the patient must have clear instructions and advice given to him with regard to diet, drugs and activity at home. Relevant help can be organized, such as rehousing, meals on wheels, routine visits from the Health Visitor, and the laundry service. Immediately on discharge a short period at a convalescent home may be advisable for some patients.

In this way the patient can benefit from nursing care not only during the period in hospital but also will lead a happier and more healthy life at home.

C. Diseases of the Heart

Rheumatic Fever

This is a disease of childhood and adolescence, about 90 per cent of the cases occurring between the ages of 5 and 15. The exact cause is not known but it often starts two or three weeks after a streptococcal throat infection and the rheumatic fever may be an allergic reaction of connective tissue in certain parts of the body to this organism. It is more common in temperate climates, for example in the British Isles, and its incidence is probably increased by bad housing and overcrowding. Since the Second World War there has been a striking reduction in the number of cases seen in this country, possibly due to improved living conditions or to the effect of antibiotic therapy on streptococcal infections.

Clinical Features Typically the illness starts rather suddenly with fever and pain, swelling and stiffness in one or more of the large joints of the limbs, that is, in the hip, knee, ankle, shoulder, elbow or wrist. After a day or two the pain often leaves the joint first affected and appears in another one, and as such flitting from joint to joint is very rare in patients with other types of arthritis, it is a useful pointer to the diagnosis. However, it is not a constant symptom. On the skin of the trunk a rash known as erythema marginatum may sometimes be seen: it consists of red blotches of irregular size and shape which have slightly raised edges, tend to join up with each other and come and go rather quickly.

In parts of the body where bones lie immediately under the skin—for example, the knuckles, wrists, elbows, ankles and scalp—rheumatic nodules may be found. They are not painful or tender and they can often be seen more easily than felt. It is important to search for these nodules in children with rheumatic fever, as they give an indication that the heart has probably also been affected. Examination of the blood usually shows a slight fall in the haemoglobin level, a slight increase in the number of white cells and a greatly raised erythrocyte sedimentation rate (ESR). This last test is of no help in making the diagnosis, since rapid sedimentation of the red cells occurs also in so many other diseases, but weekly tests showing a gradual return towards normal are of great value in indicating that the activity of the disease is subsiding.

In some children the rheumatic process takes a much milder and more insidious form which can easily be overlooked, though it is as likely as the more obvious type of acute rheumatic fever to be accompanied by active heart disease. Thus, about half the patients found later to be suffering from chronic rheumatic heart disease give no history of having had rheumatic fever or chorea (see p. 13).

Acute Carditis

Carditis means inflammation of the heart and occurs in some degree in the majority of patients with rheumatic fever. It should be suspected if the pulse is very rapid, particularly if the rise in the pulse-rate is out of proportion to the rise in temperature. The usual proportion is an increase of about 30 beats per minute for every degree Centigrade of rise in temperature; but in a patient with severe acute carditis the ratio may be 40 : 1 or even higher. Remember, however, that the excitement or distress of admission to hospital is often the cause of a very rapid pulse, and to overcome this source of error it is important to take the sleeping pulse-rate. Even if the heart-rate is not unduly fast the heart may be enlarged, or the discovery of certain murmurs, pericardial friction or electrocardiographic signs may enable the doctor to detect that the heart has been involved by the rheumatic process.

Some patients with rheumatic fever or chorea escape without evident damage to the heart, but if they get either of these diseases again carditis nearly always occurs. Similarly, existing rheumatic heart disease is almost invariably made worse by subsequent attacks of rheumatic fever or chorea.

Treatment and Nursing Care It has already been pointed out that the seriousness of this disease lies chiefly in the danger of carditis occurring at some time in the course of the illness which may result in chronic or valvular disease some months or years later.

The most important principle in the treatment of inflammation is rest. Bearing this in mind the nurse will appreciate how important it is to rest the heart, and all nursing care must be carried out with this aim in view, everything possible being done for the patient to prevent extra strain.

The patient should be nursed on a firm mattress; this will prevent unnecessary movement and give support to painful joints. The position is semirecumbent, the patient being supported by two or three pillows. In this position the cardiac output will be reduced and the patient will be more comfortable than lying flat and so will rest more readily. As *sweating is often profuse* cotton or flannel rather than nylon or other synthetic garments should be worn. Excessive sweating is more common in adults than in children, the sweat often having a sour smell which is noticed by the patient. In addition to the daily bathing in bed, additional sponging and changing into clean warm clothes will be necessary. Sweating is especially excessive round the head and neck, and causes a good deal of discomfort. The hair requires particular care, and a clean, cool pillow placed under the head should make the patient more comfortable. As a result of the high temperature and sweating, the tongue may be coated and dry, so that frequent mouth-washes are necessary and glycerine and borax may be applied to the tongue. The lips should be treated with lanoline or petroleum jelly. The affected joints may be extremely painful, swollen and red, and the greatest care possible must be taken when the patient's position has to be changed; sudden unexpected movement, such as knocking against the bed, may cause extreme pain and must be avoided. To relieve the pain the limbs may be supported on a pillow, and a bed-cradle should be used to take the weight of the bedclothes off the lower limbs. Immobilisation with light splints carefully applied and the application of methylsalicylate liniment and warm wool may all be tried in order to relieve the pain.

The temperature, pulse and respirations will be taken 4-hourly, the sleeping pulse being the most important. During the early stages the patient will be very thirsty, due to the high temperature and sweating. A variety of fluids should be given to encourage an adequate intake. The amount of urine passed will at first be scanty and highly coloured, but with sufficient fluid intake normal diuresis will occur. Gradually the patient will take a normal diet, but must be fed by the nurse through the period of complete rest. There may be constipation, and this is relieved by giving a small enema which will not unduly disturb the patient. Salicylates given by mouth have a specific action in reducing the temperature and relieving the joint pains, but they do not appear to limit the occurrence of carditis.

The drug is usually given in the form of soluble aspirin 140 mg/kg body weight (maximum 10 g) daily, given in divided doses 4-hourly; after 2 days the dosage is halved. If deafness, tinnitus, nausea and perhaps vomiting occur a further reduction in dosage is made. Fever and joint pains usually disappear within 2 to 3 days and the drug may be stopped after the patient has been free of symptoms for about a week. Prednisolone 40 mg per day may be given to patients who do not respond satisfactorily to the usual treatment.

Complete rest must be enforced until all evidence of activity of the disease has gone; in mild cases this may occur after a few weeks, but other patients have to be confined strictly to bed for many months. In particular, the sedimentation rate must have returned to normal before the patient is allowed to do anything for himself. Thereafter a graduated return to normal activity is permitted in easy stages, after each of which careful watch is kept for signs of recurrence of active rheumatism, such as for example fever, tachycardia or increase in the sedimentation rate. Prolonged convalescence in a warm, dry climate should follow, and for the future, predisposing causes of further attacks, such as undernourishment, overcrowding, dampness and cold, should if possible be avoided.

Penicillin should be administered throughout the illness; and because of the danger of further damage to the heart from a relapse of the rheumatic fever, sulphadimidine 0.5 g or oral phenoxymethyl penicillin 120 mg daily is given to prevent subsequent attacks, starting during convalescence and continuing for some 5 years or until the child reaches puberty.

Rheumatic Chorea (or Sydenham's Chorea)

This is known to the layman as St. Vitus' Dance. Its cause is probably the same as that of rheumatic fever, except that the pathological changes occur in the brain instead of in the joints, and identical lesions may occur in the heart in the two diseases. The child developing chorea is usually first noticed to be very restless and fidgety, and some time may elapse before it is appreciated that her jerkiness and clumsiness indicate illness rather than original sin. All four limbs may be affected or only one arm and leg (hemichorea). When the disease is at its height the *involuntary movements* are the most prominent feature; the child is constantly grimacing and making sudden, jerky and ever-varying movements of the limbs. In doubtful cases it is a useful test to ask the child to grasp one's hand, as she is unable to maintain a steady pressure and the intensity of her grip will be found to be always waxing and waning. The muscles are weak and have poor tone, so that the joints can be moved through an abnormally wide range of movement, and typically the outstretched hands are held with the wrists slightly flexed and the fingers hyperextended at the metacarpophalangeal joints.

Treatment and Nursing Care Rest is the most important part of the treatment of this disease in order to prevent or limit permanent damage to the heart. In comparison drug therapy is of minor importance. To achieve complete rest for this type of patient is not easy because of the very nature of the disease. Involuntary, unco-ordinated muscle movement, muscle weakness and severe emotional distress may be so extreme at times that the child is completely exhausted. Good nursing care is of paramount importance. The nurse will require great patience, a sympathetic understanding and a quiet and calm manner in order to gain the confidence and trust of her patient. Two nurses will be required to carry out any treatment and to prevent the child exerting herself and putting added strain on the heart. During the first few weeks of the illness as far as possible the same nurses should be responsible for the care of the child, and so a satisfactory nurse–patient relationship is established. The nurse becomes familiar with particular difficulties, and when aphasia is present will understand much more readily and anticipate the child's needs. The parents should be encouraged to visit as often as possible to read to her or interest her in other ways which will not disturb her rest. If the parents cannot do this a nurse or voluntary helper should find time to spend with the child.

Rest in bed is essential. Some children will benefit by being nursed in a single room, while others are happier and rest more readily if they are in a ward with other children, in which case they should be in a quiet corner. The cot or bed should have sides, and it will sometimes be necessary to pad these to prevent the child from injury during periods of extreme restlessness.

One or two pillows may be used, and a flannel gown should be provided. A flannelette blanket next to the patient may be necessary if she is sweating. The child will be given a daily bath in bed and warm sponging at other times, particularly last thing at night, as this will be soothing and will help to induce sleep.

The child may be emaciated, and areas over any prominences must be carefully treated to prevent sores resulting from constant friction. The hair will need frequent brushing and combing to avoid it becoming matted and tangled. Cleanliness of the mouth is important, and great care will be necessary when cleaning the teeth. The use of a bedpan often worries the child, unexpected involuntary movement may cause the contents to be upset, resulting in much emotional distress. Great care must be taken to avoid such an accident and in no circumstances must the child be made to feel in any way that it was her fault. Where there is constipation, it should be treated by giving a small enema of plain water or glycerine suppositories.

Feeding is one of the greatest problems. The child's appetite is variable and she is very conscious that she is not able to take her food like other children. In her efforts to do all she can to help she will often close her mouth as the spoon reaches her lips, and so the food is spilt and this causes acute distress. The tongue cannot be controlled satisfactorily and seems too big for her mouth, which increases feeding difficulties. It is important for the child to have sufficient nourishment, and so much time and great patience are required. Fluids should be given by attaching a piece of polythene tubing to the spout of a feeding-cup; china utensils should not be allowed until the movements are more controlled. Rarely, the swallowing reflex is lost, and tube-feeding will have to be used for a time.

The temperature, pulse and respiration will be taken and recorded 4-hourly, the sleeping pulse being of particular importance. The thermometer will be placed in the axilla or rectum and will be carefully held in place.

Drugs There is no specific drug for the treatment of chorea. When the child is very restless, sedatives are used to prevent exhaustion, the most useful being soluble aspirin 300 mg t.d.s. In addition diazepam 0.8 mg/kg daily in divided doses or chlorpromazine 0.5 mg/kg 12-hourly help to control restlessness.

By the end of three or four weeks the movements will have subsided and the child will be less agitated by trying to perform simple actions. At this stage simple exercises to encourage co-ordinated movement are allowed. Physiotherapy should be given prior to the patient getting up. When this should begin depends on the degree of cardiac involvement and the disappearance of involuntary movement. The child should go to a convalescent home for three to six months, preferably one where a graded amount of schooling can be given.

When the child returns to school there should be co-operation between the school doctor and nurse and the teaching staff to ensure that any slight relapse is recognised and treated without delay.

Chronic Rheumatic Heart Disease: Mitral Stenosis

During the healing stages of the acute inflammatory process in the heart which accompanies rheumatic fever and chorea, fibrous tissue is laid down in the parts of the heart which have been most severely affected. In most cases the mitral valve is involved, less frequently the aortic valve and rather rarely the tricuspid valve. Now, newly-formed fibrous tissue tends to undergo slow but steady contraction during the first year or two after its deposition, and it can be seen that when such shortening takes place in fibres which encircle the ring of, say, the mitral valve the size of the opening between the atrium and ventricle will inevitably be made progressively smaller. This, in a nutshell, is how mitral stenosis comes about. It is important to understand that the stenosis is not present at the time of the rheumatic fever; indeed, there may be no clinical evidence of it until many months or even years later. In time, however, the stream of blood flowing from the left atrium into the left ventricle in ventricular diastole meets such resistance at the fibrotic mitral valve that a characteristic murmur is produced, and this enables the expert with a stethoscope to diagnose mitral stenosis. At this stage the patient may well be in good health and have no symptoms at all. Eventually, however, the obstruction at the mitral valve causes blood to be dammed back under increased pressure in the left atrium, and consequently in the pulmonary veins which drain into it; the pulmonary vessels become distended with blood, and the resulting increased rigidity of the lungs hampers the respiratory movements. The patient now suffers from difficulty in breathing. Furthermore, rupture of one of the distended blood vessels in the lungs is not uncommon, and leads to spitting of blood (haemoptysis). The rise of pressure in the pulmonary veins leads inevitably to rise of pressure in the pulmonary artery, and this in turn puts more work on the right ventricle. At first the ventricle responds by undergoing hypertrophy and so increasing its power of contraction, but eventually even with this additional strength it becomes unable to pump the blood through the lungs quickly enough and the patient passes into right-sided cardiac failure (p. 6). Most patients with rheumatic heart disease reach this stage by early middle age, but with careful treatment the majority continue in a state of semi-invalidism for a number of years longer.

Nearly all patients with mitral stenosis develop atrial fibrillation (p. 3) after the disease has been established for some years, and the sudden onset of this arrhythmia causes a rapid increase in breathlessness or may precipitate actual heart failure. Fortunately, however, the ill-effects largely disappear when the patient is adequately digitalised.

A more serious complication may occur from detachment of a fragment of the clot which tends to form in the rather stagnant pool of blood in the dilated left atrium. Such a fragment (known as an embolus) is swept into the general circulation and causes plugging (embolism) of a systemic artery. Frequently the embolism occurs in one of the arteries to the brain and results in a form of stroke, usually causing weakness down one side of the body.

Another grave complication of mitral stenosis is subacute bacterial endocarditis (p. 18).

Treatment No treatment is indicated for mitral stenosis while the patient remains free of symptoms. When shortness of breath becomes troublesome, and preferably before the onset of actual congestive cardiac failure, the possibility of mitral valvotomy should be considered. In skilled hands this operation is of great benefit to suitable patients and the risks are now comparatively slight. The treatment of cardiac failure is described on p. 7.

Congenital Heart Disease

Congenital malformations of the heart may be subdivided into those which cause cyanosis and those which do not (the acyanotic group). The **cyanosis** in the first group is due to what is called a right–left shunt; a proportion of the blood entering the right side of the heart from the venae cavae takes a short cut into one of the chambers on the left side of the heart without passing through the lungs. The blood pumped into the aorta is consequently a combination of arterial and venous blood, and the patient has cyanosis which is called central. These 'blue babies' have clubbing of the fingers and toes, and in an attempt to compensate for the deficient oxygenation of the blood delivered to the tissues the red blood corpuscles and haemoglobin in the blood are greatly increased.

Fallot's tetralogy (literally Fallot's 'combination of four lesions') is the commonest variety of cyanotic congenital heart disease. A curious feature is the habit, seen in most of these children, of taking frequent rests in a squatting position. The four lesions are pulmonary stenosis, right ventricular hypertrophy, ventricular septal defect and an aorta which arises partly from the right ventricle and partly from the left ventricle. As a result of this combination of lesions the blood entering the right ventricle does not all take the normal route via the pulmonary artery into the lungs; some of it passes straight into the aorta, and some of it passes through the septal defect into the left ventricle and then into the aorta. Too little blood therefore passes through the lungs. Selected patients with this condition may be improved by Blalock's operation, which improves pulmonary blood flow by uniting a systemic artery with a pulmonary artery, or by Brock's operation, which directly relieves the pulmonary stenosis. More recently total correction of the deformity has been undertaken with relief of the stenosis and repair of the septal defect.

The **acyanotic cases** are of two types: those, such as congenital aortic stenosis, in which there is no abnormal communication between the two sides of the heart; and those, such as patent ductus arteriosus, ventricular septal defect (VSD) and atrial septal defect (ASD), in which the flow of blood in the abnormal channel between the two sides of the heart is from left to right so that the shunted blood instead of escaping oxygenation actually passes through the lungs twice. At first sight this might appear to be advantageous, but the load on the pulmonary circulation may lead to right heart failure, and bacterial endocarditis often develops in a patent ductus. To avoid this latter complication operation and ligature of the ductus is now usually advised.

Bacterial Endocarditis

The endocardium is the lining membrane of the heart and includes the heart valves. Bacterial endocarditis is due to bacteria gaining a foothold on some part of the endocardium and multiplying there. The acute variety usually occurs as a terminal incident in the course of an overwhelming infection by an organism of high virulence.

Subacute bacterial endocarditis is of greater clinical importance. In this type the organism is nearly always *Streptococcus viridans*, which is one of the bacteria found in the mouth and throat of healthy people. There it is perfectly harmless, but when it becomes established on a valve in the heart it gives rise to an illness which is almost invariably fatal after a period of months unless an intensive course of treatment with an appropriate antibiotic is given. The infection usually occurs on an aortic valve previously damaged by rheumatic fever, but in patients over 50 there may be no evidence of previous disease. It may complicate various congenital lesions including ventricular septal defect, pulmonary and aortic stenosis, persistent ductus arteriosus and bicuspid aortic valves. It may also develop on artificial valves. It is very rare in patients with syphilitic aortitis or atrial septal defect and in those with atrial fibrillation. The organism reaches the heart via the bloodstream, and as bacteria from the mouth can often be detected circulating in the blood after dental manipulations, particularly extractions, it is very important in the prevention of subacute bacterial endocarditis that patients with mitral stenosis or congenital heart disease should have penicillin 'cover' for any dental treatment.

The most constant clinical feature of the disease is persistent low-grade fever, and this diagnosis should be considered in every patient with mitral stenosis who develops a pyrexia for which there is no other obvious cause. Increasing tiredness and breathlessness are common symptoms. After the first week or two anaemia causes pallor, and slight clubbing of the fingers is often seen. From time to time small portions of the vegetations growing on the heart-valve break off, are swept into the general circulation and cause plugging (embolism) of small arteries in different parts of the body. Such an embolism lodging in a blood vessel supplying the skin causes a small, tender, red and slightly raised spot, most commonly seen in the pads of the fingers, and known as an Osler's node. Other common sites for embolism are the spleen, which becomes palpable and sometimes painful, and the kidney, where it causes an excess of red blood cells to appear in the urine.

Examination of the blood reveals mild or moderate anaemia and often a slight increase in the white cells (leucocytosis), and isolation of *Streptococcus viridans* by blood culture finally establishes the diagnosis. This organism does not grow very readily, so that several blood cultures usually have to be done before a positive result is obtained.

Fortunately the majority of patients can now be cured by giving benzylpenicillin 2.0 mega units four times daily for at least 6 weeks. If there is no response the dose is increased to 10 mega units or more daily and streptomycin 0.75 g b.d. and probenecid 0.5 g four times daily are added. The nurse must show great tact and firmness in dealing with these patients, many of whom come to dread the frequent injections and plead for them to be stopped prematurely.

Coronary Artery Disease

A. Angina Pectoris

Certain risk factors predisposing to the development of ischaemic heart disease have been identified. These are:

1 High plasma cholesterol levels and in particular a low level of High-Density Lipoprotein. These levels correlate well with the amount of saturated fat in the diet. Ideally not more than 30% of the daily calories should be provided by fat.

2 Hypertension.

3 Cigarette smoking.

4 'Type-A personality', characterised by aggression, impatience and excessive concern with punctuality.

5 Diabetes mellitus.

Obesity and lack of exercise also play some part, but are probably less important than the factors listed above.

A fatty substance known as atheroma becomes deposited in the wall of the artery, which in consequence becomes progressively narrower (see Figure on p. 21). Obstruction to the flow of blood eventually becomes so severe that when exercise increases the oxygen consumption of the heart-muscle not enough blood can get through in time to supply it. The patient therefore develops pain due to lack of oxygen in the myocardium: this is the pain we call **angina pectoris.** It is a heavy, constricting, painful sensation in the centre of the chest under the sternum, sometimes radiating down the arms or up into the neck or jaw, and it can be recognised as angina pectoris because it is brought on by effort and relieved by rest. Exposure to cold and emotional upsets also tend to induce it.

Depression and deep-seated anxiety often follow the patient's discovery that he has angina, which is very natural, since the liability to sudden death at a relatively early age is common knowledge. Great tact and human understanding are therefore needed in dealing with these patients, and the nurse can sometimes help very much by drawing the doctor's attention to groundless fears bred in the patient's mind by ignorance and ill-informed gossip. Many patients with angina pectoris in fact live full and useful lives for ten, fifteen or more years. The more strenuous forms of exertion must be prohibited, but gentle exercise insufficient to bring on pain is beneficial and should be encouraged. If the patient is overweight he will certainly benefit from a reducing diet, and cigarette-smoking should be abandoned or reduced to a minimum. Smoking undoubtedly reduces blood-flow, and some patients with angina improve remarkably after giving it up. Nitrites improve the coronary circulation and therefore relieve the pain of angina; they are best given as trinitrin tablets which the patient places under the tongue as soon as the pain comes on and allows to dissolve. Many patients use these tablets much too sparingly, fearing that they will harm the heart or lead to drug addiction, so that it is helpful to explain that no ill can come from their use and indeed that harm is more likely to follow failure to use them when they are needed. Propranolol is sometimes useful in angina by decreasing the sympathetic drive to the heart; it should not be given to patients in heart failure or those with a history of bronchial asthma.

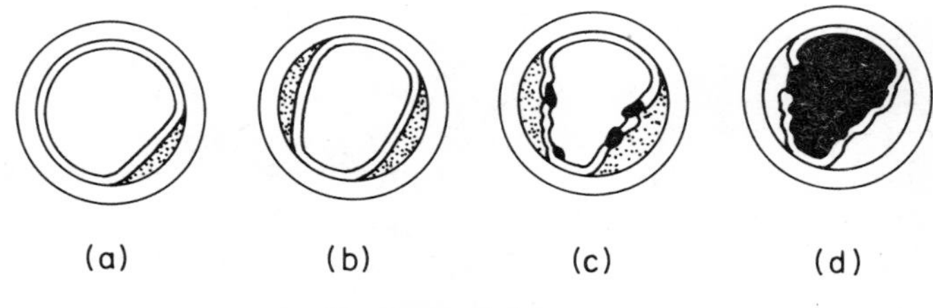

(a) (b) (c) (d)

Coronary Atheroma

(*a*) A plaque of yellow fatty atheroma has been laid down under the intimal coat of the artery. Blood flow is not impeded, and there are no symptoms.
(*b*) More atheroma has appeared and has significantly reduced the lumen; the artery now cannot accommodate the extra blood flow needed during exercise, and the patient has the pain called angina of effort.
(*c*) Roughening of the surface of the plaque of atheroma predisposes to thrombus formation.
(*d*) Eventually a clot may completely occlude the artery. This is coronary thrombosis.

B. Coronary Thrombosis

In patients with severe coronary atheroma there is always the danger that a clot may form in a narrowed and roughened part of an artery, thus suddenly and completely cutting off part of the heart-muscle (or myocardium) from its blood supply; in other words, a coronary thrombosis may occur and lead to an area of infarction in the myocardium. An infarct is a piece of tissue which has died from sudden deprivation of its blood supply (see Figure below).

When a large coronary artery is obstructed by thrombosis the patient may fall down dead; indeed, this is the commonest cause of sudden death. More often, however, the patient survives, and over a period of a few weeks the piece of dead muscle in the heart is removed by the reparative processes of the body and replaced by a simple fibrous tissue. In this way the infarcted area is eventually converted into a firm scar which, when soundly healed, may leave the wall of the heart as strong as ever. Sometimes, however, the loss of the infarcted muscle so reduces the reserve power of the heart that congestive cardiac failure occurs, and sometimes the patient is left with severe and incapacitating angina. Furthermore, in such patients there is always the risk that thrombosis may occur in another branch of a coronary artery. However, one should not be too gloomy about the prognosis, for many patients survive in reasonably good health for a decade or more after an attack of myocardial infarction.

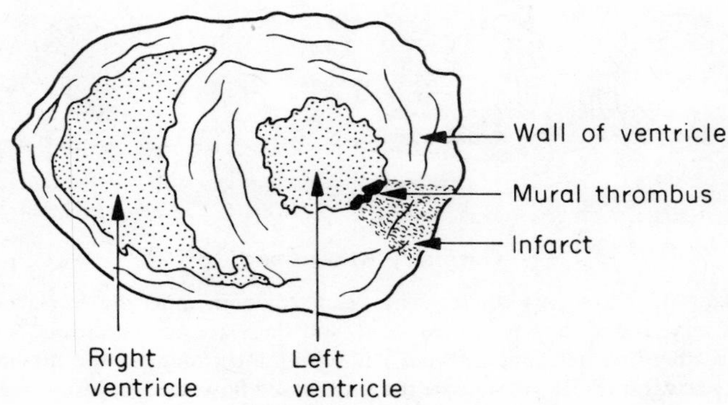

Myocardial Infarction

Coronary thrombosis leads to death from anoxia of the segment of heart muscle supplied by that artery. The dead muscle is called an infarct, and after a few weeks is replaced by firm scar tissue.

Coronary thrombosis causes a sudden severe substernal pain of the same type and distribution as angina pectoris; it can be distinguished from angina by the fact that it often comes on while the patient is at rest and, unlike angina, which is relieved by a few minutes' rest, it persists for several hours. The patient is often extremely alarmed and in fear of death and may show signs of profound shock, having a cold, clammy skin, a fast, thready pulse and a low blood pressure.

The diagnosis may sometimes be confirmed by an electrocardiogram, which may also reveal the site of the infarct in the myocardium. During the first few days the level of the transaminase enzymes in the blood rises and there may be slight fever and a raised ESR; these changes result from the damage to heart muscle.

Treatment Until the scar in the heart has healed firmly it is important to prevent any sudden rise of pressure within the ventricles which might cause rupture of the heart through the weak spot in its wall. Violent exertion and heavy lifting must therefore be avoided, but it is now usual to allow the patient out of bed after two or three days, after which in uncomplicated cases there can be a graduated return to normal activity. On admission an injection of morphine 15 or 20 mg, according to the size of the patient, will be needed to relieve his pain and mental anguish and may have to be repeated once or twice durng the first 24 hours.

Very careful observation of the patient is necessary during the acute stage; quietness is important, and he should be disturbed only for essential nursing care and treatment. Two nurses will often be needed to attend to him to save him from any unnecessary physical effort. If constipation is a cause of worry 2 glycerine suppositories may be given after 48 hours and subsequently every two or three days if necessary. Whether the patient will be allowed to be lifted out of bed to use a commode depends on the severity of the illness and the amount of distress caused to him by using a bedpan. To prevent thrombosis of the deep veins, passive exercises to the lower limbs should be given from the start and followed at a later stage by active exercises.

At one time **anticoagulant therapy** was given in an attempt to prevent the development of thrombi in the deep veins of the legs and on the endocardium, but it is now thought that the dangers of the treatment outweigh its theoretical benefits and it is seldom given except to patients with deep vein thrombosis.

Many patients are anxious or worried in the weeks following a cardiac infarct and sedation with diazepam (Valium) 2–5 mg three times daily may be useful.

Monitoring It is now realised that arrhythmias are a frequent cause of circulatory failure and death after cardiac infarction. If the patient is continuously monitored by ECG in the two or three days after infarction, these arrhythmias can be diagnosed immediately and with appropriate treatment the mortality rate can be halved. The measures used for the various arrhythmias are:

1 **Ventricular ectopics:** propranolol 10 mg q.d.s. or phenytoin 100 mg t.d.s. by mouth. Multiple ectopics are treated in the same way as:

2 **Ventricular tachycardia:** intravenous lignocaine, 50–100 mg followed if necessary by infusion at the rate of 1 mg per minute. If this fails DC shock (cardioversion) may be given.

3 **Ventricular fibrillation:** electrical defibrillation.

4 **Atrial fibrillation:** cautious digitalisation.

5 **Sinus bradycardia:** intravenous atropine 0.6 mg.

6 **Heart block:** The cardiac infarct sometimes damages the atrio-ventricular bundle so that some or all of the impulses from the sinus node fail to reach the ventricles and the heart rate becomes dangerously slow. This is corrected by the insertion of an artificial pace-maker.

If the blood pressure falls to dangerously low levels it may be helpful to raise the foot of the bed and these patients should also be given oxygen 2 litres per minute by mask (40–60 per cent).

Subsequent Management When the period of bed rest is over the patient is gradually allowed up, but he should not return to work for at least three months after the acute attack. Ideally he should then resume his normal life, but whether he will be able to do so without some modification clearly depends on the nature of his work and the completeness of his recovery.

Syphilitic Aortitis

Syphilis attacks the aorta in the tertiary stage of the disease (see p. 216), so that the symptoms do not appear until many years after the infection has been acquired. Most of the patients are men in the fifties or sixties. The essential lesion is a special type of inflammatory reaction, known as endarteritis obliterans, which cuts down the flow of blood in the tiny vessels that supply the wall of the aorta with blood. In time the powerful muscular and elastic tissue of the aorta degenerates from lack of oxygen and is replaced by simple fibrous tissue, whose oxygen requirements are much smaller. This fibrotic aorta, however, is no longer able to spring back to its resting size after each heart-beat distends it with blood; on the contrary, the fibrous wall becomes progressively stretched and the aorta becomes dilated. Usually there is a general dilatation affecting the first few inches of the aorta, but sometimes a particularly weak part of the wall balloons out into what is called a saccular aneurysm. The widening of the aorta nearly always makes it impossible for the aortic valve to prevent blood flowing back into the ventricle during diastole; in other words, it leads to aortic regurgitation. Heaping up of the lining of the aorta often occurs round the openings of the two coronary arteries in the first part of the aorta, cutting down the coronary blood-flow and causing angina pectoris (see p. 20).

The substernal pain of angina, coming on when the patient exerts himself, and relieved by rest, is therefore a common symptom of syphilitic aortitis. Other patients remain symptom-free until the strain imposed on the left ventricle by the aortic regurgitation leads to left ventricular failure (p. 5). They then suffer attacks of cardiac asthma at night and become increasingly short of breath on exertion. The course of the illness is usually rather rapidly downhill over a few years.

When an aneurysm is present it may compress important structures which lie close to it in the chest and so produce another group of symptoms and signs. It may erode its way through the chest wall, causing severe local pain and tenderness, and may eventually appear on the surface as a pulsating swelling just to the right of the sternum. More deeply placed aneurysms may compress the trachea, causing a typical brassy cough; the oesophagus, causing difficulty in swallowing; the recurrent laryngeal nerve, causing hoarseness; or the superior vena cava, causing congestion and oedema of the head and neck.

Serological tests for syphilis are usually positive. Occasionally, however, they may have reverted to negative before the disease has become clinically apparent, so that a negative test does not necessarily rule out the possibility of syphilitic aortitis.

Treatment If the syphilis is thought to be still active, an intensive course of penicillin should be given (p. 217). The treatment of left ventricular and total heart failure is described on p. 7.

Hypertension

The blood pressure is very variable in healthy people and may rise temporarily to quite high figures as the result of exertion or emotion without being in any way abnormal. Unless the patient is comfortably at rest and mentally relaxed when the blood pressure is taken, therefore, the reading may be of little value. A blood pressure of above 150/90 mmHg taken under proper conditions, should be regarded as abnormally high.

Consideration should next be given to the possible causes of this high blood pressure (or hypertension). Chronic renal disease is responsible in about 20 % of patients and would be suggested by the discovery of protein in the urine. Further investigation of the renal tract is then indicated to identify the precise kidney disease. Other rare causes of hypertension are Cushing's syndrome (p. 121); phaeochromocytoma, a tumour of the adrenal medulla which raises the blood pressure by secreting large amounts of adrenaline into the blood; Conn's syndrome, due to an adrenal tumour which secretes large amounts of aldosterone so that too much sodium is retained in the body and too little potassium; and co-arctation of the aorta, a congenital stricture of the aorta resection of which cures the hypertension. The contraceptive pill sometimes raises the blood pressure, which however returns to normal when the pill is stopped.

Essential Hypertension

In the great majority of patients with high blood pressure, however, none of the above causes is found and a diagnosis of essential hypertension has to be made. The cause of this disease is not known, but heredity is an important factor and the family history usually reveals that the patient's father or mother has also had a raised blood pressure. There are two varieties or stages:

1 **Malignant hypertension** is characterised by severe retinal changes, particularly swelling of the optic nerve itself (papilloedema), which may cause blindness; damage to the kidneys, revealed by proteinuria; and an extremely high blood pressure, the diastolic reading being usually above 140 mmHg. This type is seen mainly in men of early middle age, and in the absence of treatment death usually occurs within two years.

2 **Benign essential hypertension** is common in both sexes. The prognosis is rather better in women, many of whom live their allotted span without ever suffering serious symptoms. Common complaints of heavy throbbing headaches in the early morning, felt particularly at the back of the head, and faintness or dizziness on sudden movement. The high pressure in the aorta puts more work on the left ventricle, so that many patients eventually develop left ventricular failure (p. 5). The high pressure also increases wear and tear in the arteries, and there is therefore rather a high incidence of cerebral haemorrhage and cerebral thrombosis.

Treatment For the milder cases no treatment is needed; indeed it is usually wise not to reveal to the patient that the blood pressure is abnormal, since the effects of chronic anxiety are often worse than the disease.

General Measures Correction of obesity may result in a very satisfactory fall in blood pressure and in view of the very high incidence of coronary disease in hypertensives the patient should also be urged to stop smoking. For the same reason hyperlipidaemia if present should be treated, particularly by a diet low in saturated fat. Many of these patients are very anxious and require reassurance and perhaps sedation by diazepam 2 mg t.d.s.

Drug Treatment There are many drugs which lower blood pressure and the choice depends to some extent on the personal experience and preference of the physician. Except in severe cases it is usual to start with a diuretic such as bendrofluazide 2.5–5 mg daily; if the blood pressure remains too high a beta blocker (which reduces the sympathetic drive to the heart) is then added. Suitable beta blockers are propranolol 80 mg b.d. or atenolol 100 mg daily. It should be noted that beta blockers should not be given to patients in heart failure or with a history of asthma and that long-term use of thiazide diuretics may lead to diabetes. Other drugs in current use include hydrallazine 25 mg t.d.s., which reduces blood pressure by dilating the arterioles, and prazosin 0.5 mg t.d.s., which has a dilating effect on both arteries and veins. These are powerful drugs and patients should be warned that the first dose of prazosin may cause collapse from sudden fall in blood pressure.

Heart Disease and Pregnancy

Pregnancy produces a number of changes in the circulation which throw an increased strain on the heart and which may be wrongly interpreted as evidence of heart disease.

These changes begin during the second month of pregnancy, increase until about the thirty-second week and then diminish. The chief changes are:

(1) An increase in cardiac output.
(2) Some retention of sodium and water.

Clinically there is tachycardia, a full pulse and warm, flushed and pulsating extremities. There may be some ankle oedema, although this may also be a sign of toxaemia. The apex beat is rather forcible and may in the later months of pregnancy be displaced a little to the left. The jugular venous pressure is slightly raised. The increased cardiac flow produces pulmonary and aortic systolic murmurs. A physiological third heart sound is not uncommon due to rapid ventricular filling.

Fitness for Pregnancy The decision as to whether a patient with heart disease is fit for pregnancy is not always easy and when there is any doubt expert advice should be sought.

Generally speaking the following rules will be found useful:

(1) Patients with no symptoms or evidence of cardiac enlargement will usually go through a pregnancy without trouble.

(2) Patients who have had heart failure or who have severe effort intolerance should be advised against pregnancy; if they have already conceived, the pregnancy should be terminated in the first three months.

(3) The middle group present the main difficulty. This includes those with moderate dyspnoea on effort and some cardiac enlargement. Each of these cases will have to be judged on its own merits.

Cardiac Surgery and Pregnancy If the patient has some lesion which can be corrected surgically this should be done before pregnancy or, if the patient is already pregnant, within the first three months.

General Management during Pregnancy All patients with heart disease should be carefully observed by both physician and obstetrician.

Patients who have symptoms before pregnancy or those who develop some dyspnoea during pregnancy must have a full night's rest and in addition should rest during the afternoon. The earliest signs of cardiac failure are the development of pulmonary congestion with râles at the bases of the lungs and X-ray evidence of congestion. Filling of the neck veins and the presence of slight ankle oedema are often misleading as these may occur normally in pregnancy.

If failure develops it should be treated in the usual way (p. 7).

Management of Labour In most patients natural delivery assisted perhaps by forceps in the second stage is quite satisfactory. Caesarian section is rarely required except perhaps in co-arctation of the aorta where there is a risk of rupture.

Postpartum Period Rest is important in the postpartum period and the long-term problem of looking after a child and a home must be considered before embarking on a further pregnancy.

Mitral Stenosis in Pregnancy The vast majority of patients with heart disease and pregnancy have rheumatic heart disease, usually mitral stenosis.

The main danger in these patients is the rapid development of pulmonary congestion with attacks of pulmonary oedema, which may be fatal. This usually starts early in pregnancy and is an indication for an emergency mitral valvotomy. In addition, atrial fibrillation may start in pregnancy and produce a rapid onset of cardiac failure.

2

Disorders of the Blood and Lymphatic System

Anatomy and Physiology

Blood contains three types of cell: red blood corpuscles (or erythrocytes), white blood corpuscles (or leucocytes) and platelets (or thrombocytes). These cells are manufactured in bone-marrow and normally the speed of production is regulated to ensure that just sufficient numbers of each type of cell are delivered into the blood each day to replace those which have worn out and have been removed.

The main function of the red cells is to carry oxygen from the lungs and deliver it to all parts of the body; they can do this because of the remarkable ability of the haemoglobin they contain to combine with oxygen and then give it up again. In order to turn out plenty of normal new red cells the bone-marrow needs (in addition to other ingredients) adequate supplies of vitamin B12 and folic acid for the proper development of the red-cell envelopes, and enough iron for the haemoglobin which it puts into the envelopes. Small amounts of thyroid hormone (thyroxin), vitamin C (ascorbic acid) and copper are also required for efficient red-cell production. The life of each red cell in the circulation is about 120 days. At the end of this time cells of the reticulo-endothelial system (which are found in the spleen, liver and bone-marrow) break up and dispose of the worn-out red-cell envelope and split the haemoglobin into an iron-containing part and a non-iron-containing part. The former is returned to the bone-marrow to be built into haemoglobin for new red cells; the latter constitutes the bile pigment which circulates in the blood and is removed by the liver (see p. 92).

The white blood cells are an important part of the body's defences against various types of infection. The platelets are an essential part of the clotting mechanism which seals off the hole and stops the bleeding from an injured blood vessel.

Anaemia

Definition Anaemia is a condition of diminished oxygen-carrying capacity of the blood due to a reduction in the numbers of red cells or in their content of haemoglobin, or both.

Causes Anaemia may be due to:

1 Loss of a large quantity of blood as a result of serious bleeding from any part of the body.

2 Shortage in the bone-marrow of any of the ingredients, mentioned above, which are necessary for the manufacture of normal red cells.

3 Abnormally rapid destruction (or haemolysis) of the red cells circulating in the blood.

4 Partial or complete closing down of the bone-marrow factory (aplastic anaemia).

Symptoms and Signs of Anaemia The symptoms and signs due to diminished oxygen-carrying capacity of the blood are common to all types of anaemia. They include general tiredness, shortness of breath on exertion, giddiness, headache, pallor (especially pallor of the mucous membranes), palpitations, oedema of the ankles, and occasionally in elderly people angina pectoris (see p. 20).

Anaemia due to Haemorrhage

Immediately after the loss of up to a litre of blood, a blood count shows a normal number of red cells with a normal haemoglobin content, but within a few hours the remaining blood is diluted by tissue fluid equivalent in volume to the blood which has been lost, and now a blood count shows a severe and equal reduction in red cells and haemoglobin percentage. If no further bleeding takes place and the patient is otherwise healthy the bone-marrow increases its output of normal red cells, and within a week or two the blood count is restored to normal. A normal person contains in his body, however, reserve stores of iron which are only sufficient for the replacement of about two litres of blood, so that if bleeding continues until more than this amount has been lost the bone-marrow runs out of iron and has to produce new red cells which show signs of iron deficiency.

Iron-deficiency Anaemia

The main cause of iron-deficiency anaemia, therefore, is chronic haemorrhage; and the condition is particularly common in women during the reproductive period of life because of the blood they lose in menstruation and childbirth. Other factors leading to a deficiency of iron in the body are a diet poor in iron-containing foods, such as meat and green vegetables, and impairment of iron absorption as a result of gastrectomy or one of the malabsorption syndromes such as coeliac disease or gluten enteropathy.

In addition to the usual symptoms and signs of anaemia, patients

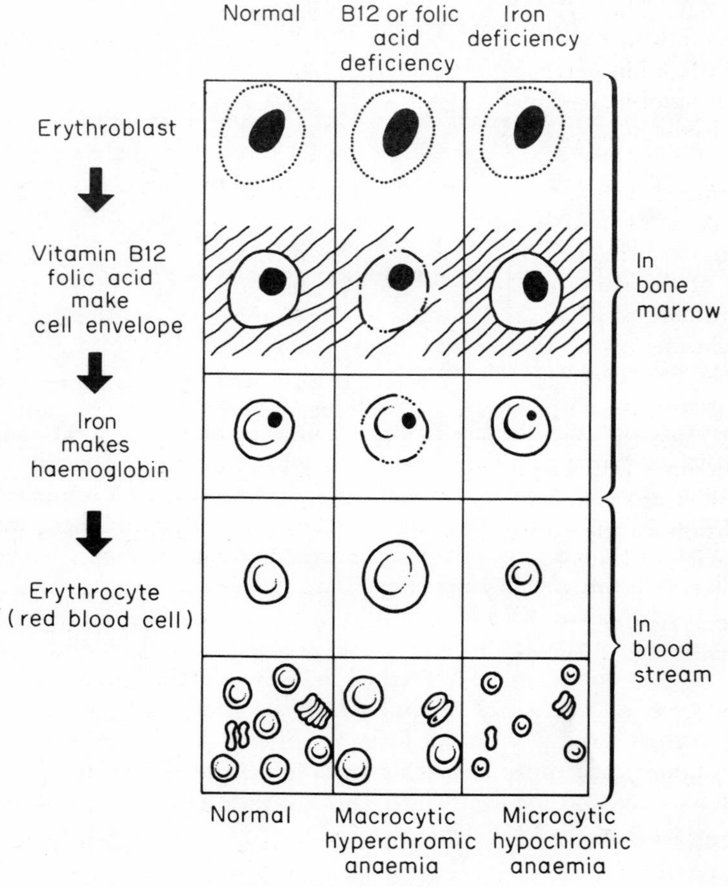

(*a*) Normal. Vitamin B12 and folic acid lead to maturation of adequate numbers of red cells, which are filled with iron-containing haemoglobin.

(*b*) Lack of vitamin B12 or folic acid: too few, immature (and therefore larger) red cells, which are overfilled with haemoglobin: a macrocytic, hyperchromic anaemia.

(*c*) Iron deficiency: plenty of red cells, but so little haemoglobin to put in them that they are small pale cells: a microcytic, hypochromic anaemia.

with iron deficiency often have brittle, spoon-shaped nails (koilonychia) and a very smooth tongue. Difficulty in swallowing (dysphagia) may occur in severe cases and completes the picture of the Plummer–Vinson syndrome (Paterson Brown–Kelly syndrome).

Iron is an essential part of the haemoglobin molecule, and when it is in short supply the bone-marrow has to put less haemoglobin into each new red cell it produces. There is no shortage of red-cell envelopes, so that the number of new red cells is approximately normal. The typical blood count therefore shows very little reduction in red blood corpuscles but a considerable reduction in haemoglobin percentage; and since each red cell contains too little haemoglobin, it is small in size (or microcytic) and deficient in colour (or hypochromic).

Treatment Since iron deficiency is usually the result of blood loss, the cause of the latter must first be investigated and treated. Apart from excessive uterine bleeding (or menorrhagia), the commonest site of the haemorrhage is the alimentary tract, and appropriate treatment may have to be given for haemorrhoids, peptic ulcer, or carcinoma of the stomach or colon.

Next the iron deficiency is corrected. This can usually be done by giving iron by mouth in the form of ferrous sulphate tablets (200 mg); the dose is one or two tablets three times daily, and sometimes improved iron absorption and better clinical response result if ascorbic acid 50 mg two or three times daily is given in addition. Some patients complain that iron by mouth upsets the stomach or bowels, and for them tab. ferrous gluconate 0.65 g may be tried in place of the ferrous sulphate. If the haemoglobin percentage does not rise satisfactorily with this treatment a suitable preparation of iron may be given by injection.

Anaemias due to Vitamin B12 Deficiency

Pernicious Anaemia (Addison's Anaemia) This is primarily a disease of the stomach, which becomes atrophic and fails to secrete the normal gastric juices. It does not occur before the age of about 30, so that the patients are all middle-aged or elderly. As a result of the failure of gastric function the vitamin B12 in the food is not absorbed and the bone-marrow is therefore deprived of this factor, which is essential for the development of normal red blood corpuscles. Another consequence of the gastric atrophy is that the stomach contains no hydrochloric acid. The diagnosis is confirmed by examining a specimen of bone-marrow obtained by inserting a needle into the sternum or iliac crest; by finding a low serum B12 level (normal 200–800 pg); or by the Schilling test, in which radioactive B12 is given by mouth and the proportion of it absorbed is estimated from the amount recovered from the urine.

When vitamin B12 is lacking the bone-marrow cannot produce enough normal red-cell envelopes, but it is not short of haemoglobin. It therefore puts more haemoglobin than normal into each available envelope. The typical blood count consequently shows a great reduction in the numbers of red blood corpuscles and a much smaller reduction in the haemoglobin percentage; and as each red cell contains an excess of haemoglobin it is large in size (macrocytic) and has increased colour (hyperchromic). These large cells are more fragile than normal ones, and their abnormally rapid breakdown (or haemolysis) in the circulation liberates an excess of bilirubin into the blood and gives the patient a typical pale lemon-yellow colour. The tongue is often sore and smooth.

Adequate supplies of vitamin B12 appear to be necessary also for the health of certain parts of the nervous system, and patients with pernicious anaemia may develop subacute combined degeneration of the spinal cord (see p. 152).

Treatment Pernicious anaemia can be corrected by intramuscular injections of vitamin B12 as cyanocobalamin (cytamen) or hydroxocobalamin (Neocytamen). There is a good deal of individual variation in dosage, but average doses are 100–1000 μg daily until the blood count is normal, followed by the same amount every 2–4 weeks for maintenance. Treatment has to be continued for the rest of the patient's life, and its effectiveness should be checked by blood counts every 2 or 3 months. No patient with pernicious anaemia should be allowed to leave hospital until the importance of these points has been made quite clear to him, for unless his blood count is kept well up to normal there is grave danger that the development of subacute combined degeneration may do irreparable damage to his spinal cord.

Other Macrocytic Anaemias, very similar to pernicious anaemia, are also due to lack of adequate supplies of vitamin B12, or folic acid, or both of these factors, in the bone-marrow. In parts of the world where malnutrition is common, dietary deficiency of folic acid or vitamin B12 causes nutritional (sometimes called tropical) macrocytic anaemia; failure of absorption of the same factors often causes macrocytic anaemia in diseases of the intestine such as sprue and gluten enteropathy; and occasionally a macrocytic anaemia, which usually responds to tablets of folic acid 10 mg daily, occurs for reasons unknown during pregnancy.

Haemolytic Anaemia

There are two main reasons why the red cells may break down (haemolyse) before their normal life of about 120 days:

1 There may be an inherited fragility of the red cells, as in **Familial Acholuric Jaundice.** In this disease the tendency for the red cells to break down increases at certain times, and at these haemolytic crises the patient rapidly develops the symptoms and signs of anaemia. He also becomes jaundiced because bilirubin is liberated from the haemoglobin of the haemolysed cells. Removal of the enlarged spleen is usually a very effective form of treatment.

Thalassaemia occurs in people of Mediterranean origin. It is due to an inherited metabolic fault leading to continued production of foetal haemoglobin. The major form is seen in homozygotes, who usually die in childhood from haemolytic anaemia; splenectomy may reduce the need for transfusion, but there is no generally effective treatment. The minor form, seen in heterozygotes, is usually symptomless.

2 In certain malignant and infective diseases, and sometimes for unknown reasons, a substance known as a haemolysin appears in the blood and attacks the red cells, causing an **Acquired Haemolytic Anaemia.** The haemolysins in the blood can be demonstrated by the **Coomb's test** and the abnormal haemolysis can be controlled by steroid therapy.

Aplastic Anaemia

This is the result of destruction of those cells in the bone-marrow which produce the red cells, the white cells and the platelets. Sometimes this closing-down in the bone-marrow factory affects only the department responsible for white-cell production; this variety is known as agranulocytosis (literally 'absence of the granular cells'). Death or destruction of these vital blood-making cells is sometimes a toxic reaction to certain drugs, notably amidopyrin, sulphonamides, heavy metals such as gold or arsenic, thiouracil, chloramphenicol or tridione; or to certain industrial poisons such as benzol and its derivatives. It may also result from excessive exposure to X-rays or radio-active materials. Frequently, however, the cause is not known (idiopathic aplastic anaemia).

Failure in production of red cells causes symptoms and signs of anaemia; diminished or absent output of white cells impairs the body's defences against infection, leading to painful ulceration of the throat and fever; and scarcity of platelets in the blood causes purpura and bleeding from different parts of the body.

Treatment consists in removal of the cause, if possible; fresh blood transfusion repeated as often as necessary for the correction of the anaemia; and the administration of penicillin or other suitable antibiotic to combat infection. Sometimes the affected bone-marrow cells eventually recover and the patient is restored to normal health.

Leukaemia

Leukaemia is a disease characterised by abnormal hyperplasia (over-growth) of the cells responsible for producing the white blood corpuscles. Its cause is not known, but it is generally regarded as a variety of cancer, and the risk of developing it is greatly increased by exposure to excessive radiation: many of the survivors of the Nagasaki and Hiroshima atomic explosions, for example, subsequently developed leukaemia. In this country the number of cases per million of the population has almost doubled in the last 20 years, but it is still fortunately a rare disease.

Leukaemia is classified, according to the type of leucocyte affected, into:

(1) Lymphatic leukaemia, in which the precursor cells of the lymphocytes are involved.

(2) Myeloid leukaemia, affecting the precursors of the granulocyte or polymorphonuclear leucocytes.

(3) Monocytic leukaemia.

In many ways the clinical classification into **acute leukaemia** and **chronic leukaemia** is more important.

Acute Leukaemia

Acute lymphatic leukaemia, acute myeloid leukaemia and acute monocytic leukaemia present identical clinical pictures, so that one description suffices for all. Nearly all the patients are children, adolescents or young adults, though sometimes an older patient with chronic leukaemia has a terminal acute exacerbation. Boys are affected more often than girls. The onset is usually sudden, with high fever, sore throat and bleeding from the mouth, nose or elsewhere, and it quickly becomes clear that the child is gravely ill. The diagnosis is established by the blood count and by examination of the marrow (a sample of which is obtained by puncture of the sternum or iliac crest). Anaemia rapidly becomes severe and is relieved only very temporarily by blood transfusion. The course is rapidly downhill and in the absence of treatment death usually occurs in a few weeks. Remission can now be induced in the great majority of these patients by giving prednisolone with various combinations of cytotoxic drugs, and the response to treatment of children with acute lymphoblastic leukaemia in particular is one of the most spectacular medical advances of recent years; quite a high proportion of patients with this formerly fatal disease can now be cured.

Chronic Leukaemia

Chronic Lymphatic Leukaemia is nearly always seen in men of late middle age. The patient complains of slowly developing tiredness, due to the associated anaemia, and the spleen, liver and lymph-nodes in the neck, axillae and elsewhere are found to be enlarged. The white count typically shows enormous numbers of lymphocytes. Although the disease is always fatal, many patients live for 10 years or more.

Chronic Myeloid Leukaemia occurs mainly between early adult life and middle age and is rather commoner in men than women. Slowly progressive tiredness due to anaemia is usually the presenting symptom; the spleen becomes even larger than in chronic lymphatic leukaemia, but there are no palpable lymph-nodes. The white count typically shows greatly increased numbers of polymorph leucocytes, a proportion of which are abnormally primitive, and marrow examination finally establishes the diagnosis. The course of the disease does not usually extend over more than two or three years.

Treatment of Leukaemia The object of treatment is the destruction of abnormal leucocytes and the suppression of abnormal leucocyte proliferation. Many drugs are now available which damage these rapidly dividing cells more than normal cells; they all cause severe bone marrow depression and throughout the treatment regular blood counts must be done, but by giving several of these drugs together with prednisolone at well-spaced intervals it is possible to achieve a maximum effect on the leukaemic tissue with minimal damage to healthy cells. The drugs used include chlorambucil, cyclophosphamide, busulphan, 6-mercaptopurine, methotrexate and vincristine. Ideally the treatment should be controlled by a physician with special experience in this complex and rapidly changing subject. In a few specialised units bone-marrow transplantation is being used after ablation of the malignant cells. Results are encouraging, particularly in children.

Symptomatic Treatment Transfusion is often required for anaemia in acute leukaemia and occasionally in the chronic types. Penicillin or other appropriate antibiotic is given in large doses for infective lesions in the mouth or elsewhere. In the chronic leukaemias local lesions such as painful splenomegaly may be relieved by radiotherapy.

Haemorrhagic Diseases

A tendency to abnormal bleeding may result from

1 A deficiency of blood platelets,

2 Lack of one of the various substances in the blood which are necessary for the formation of blood-clot, particularly prothrombin and antihaemophilic globulin, or

3 Some abnormality in the blood capillaries.

Groups (1) and (3) are causes of **purpura**: that is, spontaneous bleeding occurs into the skin, and often too from one or more mucous membranes. A purpuric spot in the skin can be easily recognised because it does not fade on pressure. Diseases in group (2) do not cause purpura or spontaneous bleeding, but are characterised by persistence of haemorrhage after injury.

1. Thrombocytopenia (deficiency of blood platelets)

Lack of sufficient numbers of circulating platelets occurs in a disease of unknown cause, called idiopathic thrombocytopenia, and is sometimes the result of various diseases of the bone-marrow which destroy the platelet-forming megakaryocytes. Important examples of such diseases are leukaemia and aplastic anaemia, and obviously in this group of causes the deficiency of platelets is only a small incident in the course of the primary disease.

Idiopathic thrombocytopenia is a rare disease usually seen in children or young adults, and is characterised by episodes of skin purpura and bleeding from such sites as the nose, the uterus and the alimentary tract. The blood platelet count is very low. Splenectomy is often a successful form of treatment, but it may be dangerous when the disease is in an acute phase, and the effect of repeated blood transfusions and a course of prednisolone tablets should be tried first.

2. *Coagulation Defects*

The formation of a normal clot when blood is shed is an extremely complex process and is essential for the arrest of haemorrhage after injury. A number of different substances must be present in blood before it will clot; deficiency of any one of them causes a coagulation defect (i.e. poor clot formation), with consequent persistence of bleeding after injury. Two of the most important of these essential clotting factors are prothrombin and antihaemophilic globulin.

Prothrombin Deficiency Prothrombin is manufactured in the liver from vitamin K. Vitamin K is manufactured by certain bacteria in the intestine and is also present in a number of vegetable foods; it is not absorbed properly in the absence of bile salts. Clinical prothrombin deficiency is seen mainly in two groups of patients: newborn babies in whose intestines the vitamin K-forming organisms have not yet become established (haemorrhagic disease of the newborn); and patients with obstructive jaundice whose intestine contains no bile salts. The former variety can be largely prevented by giving vitamin K 5 mg intramuscularly daily to the expectant mother for a few days before delivery. Patients with obstructive jaundice should receive similar treatment, particularly if any surgical operation is contemplated, otherwise serious haemorrhage is liable to occur.

Haemophilia Haemophilia is due to lack of an essential clotting factor known as antihaemophilic globulin. The disease is hereditary and occurs only in males, being transmitted to them by clinically normal females. The most important symptoms are persistent bleeding after cuts, abrasions or dental extractions, and bleeding into joints (haemarthroses), which may occur after trivial injury. Operations on haemophiliacs are always extremely dangerous, probably carrying a mortality in the region of 50 per cent.

Treatment consists of repeated fresh blood transfusion or preferably daily IV injections of anti-haemophilic globulin until the bleeding stops.

3. Haemorrhage due to Capillary Defects

Purpura is occasionally seen in patients with severe infection or malignant disease, probably from some obscure effect on the blood capillaries.

Anaphylactoid purpura is another variety in which the extravasation of blood into the skin and other tissues appears to be an allergic phenomenon. There are two clinical types. In Schönlein's purpura, oedema and bleeding into the skin are accompanied by swelling of joints; in Henoch's variety there is skin purpura and abdominal pain from bleeding into the wall of the intestine.

Hodgkin's Disease

This is a disease of adolescents and young adults and is commoner in men. The tissue changes are probably initiated by a viral infection, but the clinical picture is that of a progressive malignant disease. The first symptom is usually the painless enlargement of a group of superficial lymph-nodes, often in the neck. As the disease progresses, other groups of nodes become involved, including those in the mediastinum and abdomen, and the liver and spleen become enlarged as a result of infiltration with 'Hodgkin' tissue.

Less often there is involvement of other structures such as the skin and the nervous system. An interesting and helpful symptom is pain after the taking of alcohol. Bouts of fever occur in some cases, and some anaemia always develops in the later stages. The disease used to be almost invariably fatal, but modern therapy directed by a specialist in oncology brings the hope of cure. Of patients given radiotherapy for disease localised to one group of nodes over half survive for 5 years and a third for 15 years. Young women have the best outlook. The administration of a combination of cytotoxic drugs with prednisolone in a series of short courses, separated by intervals which give the healthy cells of the body time to recover, is now giving promising results and is particularly indicated for patients with generalised disease. A typical course for an adult is:

Mustine 6 mg/m^2 IV	Days 1 and 7
Vinblastine 10 mg IV	Days 1, 7 and 14
Procarbazine 100 mg orally	Days 1–14 inclusive
Prednisolone 40 mg orally	Days 1–14 inclusive

The courses are repeated at four-week intervals to a total of six courses. Smaller doses must be given if the white count is low.

3
The Respiratory System

Anatomy and Physiology

For descriptive purposes it is convenient to subdivide the respiratory system into the upper respiratory tract, consisting of the nose, nasopharynx and larynx, and the lower respiratory tract, comprising the trachea, bronchi and lungs. The lining membrane of the air passages has a rich blood supply which enables it to warm and moisten the inspired air. A film of sticky mucus covers the whole respiratory tract from the nose to the smallest bronchi, and is kept continuously moving upwards away from the lungs by the sweeping action of the tiny hair-like cilia projecting from the mucous membrane; this is a most effective filter for removing particles of dust from the air before it reaches the lungs. The irregularity of the nasal cavity and the accessory air sinuses which open into it increase the area of mucous membrane with which the air comes into contact, and so make the warming and filtering more efficient; on the other hand, swelling of the mucous membrane readily obstructs drainage of secretions from the sinuses and so may predispose to sinusitis. Another important defence mechanism is the cough reflex, which is elicited as soon as any foreign material threatens the approach to the larynx.

Types of Cough and Sputum

A cough is made possible by closure of the glottis during a sharp expiration, so that a high air pressure is built up in the trachea and bronchi; then sudden opening of the glottis is followed by explosive discharge of air from the air passages, tending to remove collections of mucus or foreign bodies and producing the characteristic barking noise. Irritation of nerve-endings in the larynx, trachea or bronchi is the trigger mechanism which fires off the cough reflex.

This irritation may be caused by inflammatory swelling of the mucous membrane itself, in patients with acute laryngitis, tracheitis or bronchitis; and as in the early stages there is no mucous exudate to be expelled, the cough is dry and unproductive. A day or two later inflammatory exudate on the surface of the mucosa elicits the cough, and small quantities of sticky, clear or whitish sputum are produced. A special variety of this type of cough occurs in **Whooping Cough.** In this disease the exudate in the air passages is particularly tough and sticky, and the patient gives a series of quickly repeated coughs during one expiratory movement in an effort to dislodge them, and then sometimes produces a 'whoop' by taking a long breath in through a partially closed glottis. Many patients never actually whoop, but the diagnosis can be made by simply hearing the typical paroxysms of rapid, barking coughs.

The presence of pus in sputum makes it yellow or greenish in colour, and since only certain bacteria are pyogenic (that is, cause pus to form), the simple observation of this colour in the sputum gives important diagnostic information. Yellow, purulent nasal secretions are seen after the first few days of the common cold, due to invasion of the nasal mucosa by secondary organisms, and for the same reason purulent sputum is usually produced by patients who have passed the initial stages of acute bronchitis, tracheitis and laryngitis.

Yellow or green purulent sputum is also expectorated by patients with **bronchiectasis,** but in much larger quantities, usually several ounces a day. This sputum collects during the night in the dilated bronchi, which are the essential pathological feature of this disease, and only when the patient gets out of bed in the morning is the cough reflex elicited by the accumulated secretions flowing on to areas of healthy bronchial mucosa. This is why bronchiectatics usually cough up a great deal of sputum first thing in the morning. Sometimes the sputum is not only purulent but very offensive in smell, from the action of putrefactive bacteria, and haemorrhage from the inflamed bronchial mucosa occasionally causes it to be bloodstained. Enzymes from pus-cells in sputum liquefy the mucus, so that purulent sputum is much more fluid than other types, and when bronchiectatic sputum, for example, is allowed to stand in a glass vessel it can be seen to separate into three layers. These are an upper layer of froth, then a more or less clear fluid layer and at the bottom a thick layer of pus and other debris.

A **bronchial carcinoma** presses on the mucous membrane of the bronchus in which it is growing and causes a cough, which is at first dry and unproductive. When it grows bigger, however, it partially obstructs the upward passage of the film of mucus on the surface of the mucosa; a stagnant pool of secretions therefore collects below the tumour and becomes infected, so that a little mucopurulent sputum is now expectorated. Erosion of small blood vessels by the carcinoma is common, and blood-streaking of the sputum is therefore very characteristic of this disease.

Spitting of blood (haemoptysis) is also an important symptom of **pulmonary tuberculosis,** and this is the diagnosis one should suspect when a young adult who has previously been in good health suddenly coughs up a fairly large quantity of blood. It is not usually streaking of the sputum with blood, as in patients with bronchial carcinoma, but the expectoration of an ounce or more of bright red blood. Tuberculosis is not a pyogenic infection, so that unless there is secondary infection the sputum contains no pus: it is therefore not yellow in colour, offensive in smell or fluid in consistence, but clear or white and very sticky, so that it remains in separate lumps in the sputum mug.

Patients with **lobar pneumonia** at the stage of resolution cough up sputum containing specks of altered blood which give it a rusty colour seen in no other disease.

Cardiac asthma (p. 6) is due to acute engorgement of the lungs with blood, and as this may lead to exudation of oedema fluid into the alveoli, the attack sometimes ends with the expectoration of a large quantity of clear, frothy sputum. In **bronchial asthma,** however, the sputum comes up in firm, whitish pellets: these can sometimes be unravelled in water into spiral ribbons (Curschmann's spirals) which represent casts of the bronchial tube in which they have formed.

Pain in the Chest

Pain in the chest is not always due to disease in the lungs, but may arise in the chest wall or in other organs which lie in the thorax. In the former group mention may be made of fracture or secondary deposit of carcinoma in a rib, which cause severe local pain and tenderness; in the latter coronary thrombosis (p. 21) and hiatus hernia (p. 82) are common examples. The most important pulmonary cause of pain in the chest is **acute dry pleurisy.** This pain is sharp and stabbing in character and is made worse by deep breathing or coughing; the pain is felt in the part of the chest which lies over the area of inflammation in the pleura, but when the diaphragmatic pleura (which lines the under surface of the lungs) is involved the pain is referred to the tip of the shoulder. This is because the diaphragmatic pleura receives its sensory nerve supply from the same spinal nerve-roots which supply the skin over the shoulder.

Types of Respiration

Air enters the lungs as a result of the descent of the diaphragm (diaphragmatic respiration) or expansion of the chest (costal respiration). These are both powerful muscular movements, and in quiet breathing each plays a variable part in different people: thus, in most men respiration is mainly diaphragmatic in type and in most women it is mainly costal. By contrast, expiration is a much less powerful movement, and results from the elastic recoil of the lungs themselves, and from relaxation of the diaphragm and of the muscles of the chest wall. The consequence is that when there is any obstruction to the free passage of air through the bronchial tubes, as for example in bronchial asthma, expiration being weaker is impeded to a greater extent than inspiration and the lungs become more and more over-distended with air. Furthermore, this is why **asthmatic breathing** is characterised by a short gasping inspiration followed by a prolonged wheezing expiratory phase.

Another characteristic abnormality of breathing is seen in patients with **acute lobar pneumonia,** who usually have an area of acute dry pleurisy overlying the solid part of the lung. The respirations are therefore not only rapid but very shallow, inspirations being abruptly stopped, often with an audible grunt, as soon as the pleuritic pain is felt. After a short pause the patient breathes out and then at once starts the next inspiration. In addition to the breathing being rapid and shallow, therefore, it has an altered rhythm, since in health the pause between breaths comes between expiration and the following inspiration, not between inspiration and expiration.

In **diabetic coma** very deep breathing ('air hunger') occurs as a result of stimulation of the respiratory centre in the brain by ketone bodies in the blood. Similarly, in the later stages of **uraemia** accumulation of acid in the blood leads to deep hissing respiration.

Cheyne-Stokes breathing is described on p. 7.

Diseases of the Upper Respiratory Tract

Coryza (The common cold)

Coryza is due to invasion of the mucous membrane of the nose and nasopharynx by a virus, and spread of the infection occurs particularly in crowded places such as buses, trains and cinemas. Sudden changes of temperature seem to predispose some people to catch a cold. After the sneezing and profuse watery nasal discharge of the first day or two, secondary infection with pyogenic bacteria often occurs and the secretion then becomes thick and yellow. Infection may spread:

1 To the accessory nasal sinuses. Acute sinusitis causes fever and severe headache or pain in the face, and localised tenderness may be found over the frontal or maxillary sinuses. After the acute stage has passed the patient is often left with chronic sinusitis, characterised by persistent purulent discharge and a tendency to acute exacerbations of symptoms whenever he acquires a fresh cold.

2 To the middle ear (via the Eustachian tube) causing acute otitis media with fever, deafness and severe earache.

3 To the lower respiratory tract causing tracheitis, bronchitis or bronchopneumonia.

Treatment There is no specific treatment for the common cold, but a day or two in bed at the onset usually cuts short the course and prevents complications. It also helps to limit spread of the infection.

Hay Fever and Perennial Rhinitis

Hay fever and perennial rhinitis are allergic disorders characterised by bouts of sneezing, a profuse watery nasal discharge and smarting and watering of the eyes. Hay fever is due to sensitivity to grass pollen and occurs therefore only during the months May to August; perennial rhinitis is due to sensitivity to a variety of materials, such as house dust, and it therefore often occurs throughout the whole year. Skin testing may help in revealing the sensitivity, and a course of desensitising injections may then be given, but many patients are relieved of their symptoms more simply by antihistamine tablets. It may be necessary to try several antihistamine preparations in various doses until satisfactory relief is obtained without too much of the drowsiness which these tablets tend to induce. Nasal insufflation of beclomethasone dipropionate (Beconase) is often very effective and does not incur the risks of systemic steroid therapy.

Influenza

Influenza is a virus infection whose severity varies greatly in different epidemics; fortunately it has not in recent years shown anything like the virulence of the great outbreak of 1918, which caused innumerable deaths throughout the world. The illness starts abruptly one or two days after exposure to infection with fever, headache and pains in the back and limbs. The face is flushed, the eyes are suffused and there is usually a reduction in the white cells in the blood (leucopenia). In mild cases recovery may occur within a week, though weakness and depression often persist for a considerable time thereafter; or infection may spread to cause laryngitis, tracheitis or bronchitis, and the latter occasionally develops into bronchopneumonia, which may be fatal.

Treatment and Nursing Care The majority of patients will be nursed in their own homes. They should be isolated in a quiet, well-ventilated room and remain in bed until the temperature has been normal for two or three days.

The aching of limbs and back and headache will be relieved by aspirin 600 mg or tab. codeine co. given three times a day. The patient will have no desire for food while fever is present, but must be encouraged to drink 3 litres of fluid a day, which will help to reduce the temperature and eliminate the toxins. If any signs of pulmonary congestion occur, penicillin therapy must commence. An expectorant mixture may be given, or linctus codeine at night will relieve an irritating cough.

Sweating may be profuse, and warm blankets, bed linen and night attire should be ready for changing the patient as required. When pyrexia has subsided, the patient will feel weak and listless. The degree of weakness and depression bears no relationship to the length of time spent in bed. There should be a gradual increase in the time the patient is up each day.

The appetite will be poor and the patient will have to be tempted to eat small amounts of nourishing food, gradually increasing to a normal diet. The period of convalescence should be adequate to prevent a relapse and overcome the depression which may persist. Excessive exercise should be avoided. It may be difficult for the above treatment to be carried out, particularly for an elderly patient living alone; and if it is not possible for relatives or friends to look after the patient, the Home Help Service should be made use of and visits from the District Nurse should be arranged.

Prophylactic Treatment Unfortunately there are many strains of influenza virus and vaccines prepared from the strains prevalent at any one time frequently fail to give protection in the epidemic of the following winter. Nevertheless it is a good plan to give an annual inoculation to debilitated patients in whom an attack of influenza would be specially hazardous.

Acute Laryngitis

Acute laryngitis occurs as a complication of the common cold or of one of the acute specific fevers of childhood, such as measles, or it may result from the inhalation of irritant gases. The throat is sore, the voice is at first hoarse and then reduced to a whisper and there is a dry, painful cough. In small children swelling of the mucous membrane of the larynx may cause serious obstruction to the passage of air, the condition sometimes known as 'croup'; breathing becomes noisy and laboured and alarming paroxysms of coughing occur.

Treatment and Nursing Care If the temperature is raised the patient should be in bed, in a warm room where the atmosphere is not too dry. The dryness of central heating, electric and gas fires can be prevented by some means of humidification. The patient must not talk, since his larynx needs rest. Smoking is also forbidden. Steam inhalations containing tincture benzoin co. 4 ml to half a litre boiling water, given for ten minutes three times a day, will give great relief; hot gargles and frequent hot drinks will help to reduce the inflammation. Simple remedies such as honey, glycerine and lemon will help to relieve the soreness of the pharynx. Linctus codeine 4 ml will suppress an irritating and unproductive cough.

Acute laryngitis in young children (croup) may be a very serious condition, as the airway quickly becomes obstructed by the swollen mucous membrane. The above treatment should be given, a steam tent being used in place of the inhaler. A sedative such as chloral hydrate or phenobarbitone may be necessary. The signs of laryngeal obstruction must be appreciated, as tracheotomy may have to be performed.

Chronic Laryngitis

After repeated attacks of acute laryngitis the voice may become more or less permanently weak and husky, and this chronic condition is particularly likely to occur in people given to excessive shouting. Hence the term 'clergyman's throat'; perhaps 'costermonger's throat' would be a less offensive and more accurate expression, since over-indulgence in tobacco and alcohol are other predisposing causes. Mouth-breathing due to nasal obstruction also often plays a part.

It is extremely important that the larynx of all such patients should be examined by an expert to make sure that the hoarseness and irritation in the throat are not due to a more serious cause, such as tuberculosis or carcinoma of the larynx.

Treatment The most important measure is complete rest to the voice; the patient must not be allowed to speak, perhaps for a matter of weeks. Any nasal obstruction should be corrected and tobacco and alcohol forbidden.

Diseases of the Lower Respiratory Tract

Acute Tracheitis and Bronchitis

Acute infections of the trachea and bronchi attack particularly young children and elderly people, though they may occur at any age if the general resistance of the patient has been lowered by some other cause. Some people are 'chesty': that is, they have a chronic low-grade infection somewhere in the bronchial tree which tends to flare up into acute tracheobronchitis whenever they catch a cold. Cold, damp and foggy weather predisposes to such infections, which also commonly occur as complications of the acute specific fevers of childhood.

Tracheitis causes a dry, painful cough and a sore feeling behind the sternum. When the infection spreads down to the bronchi the patient complains of tightness in the chest, wheezing and difficulty in breathing (dyspnoea). At first there is very little sticky mucoid sputum, but after a few days secondary infection with pyogenic bacteria makes it yellow (from the presence of pus) and more profuse. The height and duration of the fever and the degree of general malaise are very variable; usually the illness is a mild one, lasting perhaps a week or ten days, but in very young or weakly patients it may develop into the much more serious broncho-pneumonia.

Treatment and Nursing Care From the above account the nurse will appreciate the age groups in which acute bronchitis is most likely to be serious. The patient should be kept in a warm, even temperature, not too dry, and rest is essential. As with any feverish illness, he should be nursed in bed until the pyrexia has subsided. Breathing will be easier if he is sitting up with a warm, soft bed-jacket round the shoulders.

The hard, dry, painful cough in the early stages can be very exhausting and may interfere with sleep, which is very necessary. A warm, sweet drink may relieve the cough, but a dose of linctus codeine or a similar cough depressant may be given. Occasionally a hypnotic will be required to induce sleep.

When the sputum becomes purulent the organism present is usually *Haemophilus influenzae* and/or *Strep. pneumoniae* and amoxycillin 250 mg by mouth every 8 hours is the antibiotic of choice. Alternatives for patients allergic to penicillin are co-trimoxazole (Septrin) two tablets twice daily or erythromycin 250 mg 6-hourly.

The patient must be given plenty of fluids to drink; drinks such as hot lemon, are helpful and later he will require a light nourishing diet.

Constipation can usually be avoided by giving a mild aperient. The patient will be washed in bed for a few days, and care of the mouth is important. When the patient begins to get up, draughts and sudden changes of temperature must be avoided.

Chronic Bronchitis

Chronic bronchitis is a disease of middle-aged and elderly men. Its cause is not fully understood, but it occurs particularly in manual workers in industrial areas, and no doubt prolonged exposure to cold, damp weather and breathing heavily polluted air are partly responsible. Excessive cigarette-smoking and obesity are certainly important aggravating factors in many patients. The patient complains at first of a winter cough, which through the years becomes gradually more severe and disabling and is eventually present throughout the whole year. Progressive shortness of breath now becomes an even more urgent symptom. Damage to the lungs increases the resistance to the pulmonary blood-flow, which gives the right ventricle more work to do, so that in time many patients pass into right-sided cardiac failure ('cor pulmonale'). This is shown clinically by distended veins in the neck, an engorged and tender liver and oedema of the ankles.

Treatment The patient should be protected from the adverse influences mentioned above, so that if possible a job should be found for him which does not expose him to changeable weather or to dusty, smoky or foggy atmospheres. Smoking should be given up or reduced to a minimum and obesity corrected by careful dieting. Properly taught breathing exercises, combined with postural drainage to keep the bronchi as free of secretions as possible, not only reduce the coughing and dyspnoea but also help to prevent complications such as broncho-pneumonia and further damage to the lungs. For helping to clear the chest of sputum there is nothing better than the 'Brompton hot-water mixture': 15 ml of mist. sod. chlor. co. in a few ounces of very hot water first thing in the morning. Acute exacerbations following winter infections should be treated promptly with a full course of tetracycline or ampicillin. The treatment of heart failure is considered on p. 7.

Pneumonia

The term pneumonia implies that the affected part of the lung has become consolidated. First the alveoli are filled with an inflammatory exudate, and when this exudate coagulates the lung is converted from its normal spongy, air-containing state to a solid structure which looks and feels rather like a piece of liver.

Broncho-pneumonia is usually a complication of some disease of the bronchi, such as acute bronchitis or bronchiectasis, and consists of little patches of consolidation round the bronchi or bronchioles throughout both lungs.

Lobar pneumonia, on the other hand, is a primary infection of the lung tissue, and in its typical form causes consolidation of the whole of one lobe.

This is the old-fashioned, but still very useful, classification of pneumonia according to the anatomical distribution of the disease in the lungs. Pneumonia can also be subdivided by reference to the infecting organism. Thus, the commonest bacterium is the pneumococcus; this usually causes a lobar pneumonia, though it may cause broncho-pneumonia in young children and in very weak or elderly people. Streptococci and staphylococci are other bacteria which cause special types of pneumonia. Certain filterable viruses (too small to be seen under the ordinary microscope) also cause pneumonia, which is usually clinically milder than the bacterial varieties.

Lobar Pneumonia

Lobar pneumonia may occur at any age, but it is commonest in young adults. Men are affected more often than women. The onset is usually sudden, perhaps with a shivering attack or rigor followed by fever, general malaise and frequently pain in the chest. The patient looks flushed and ill and the temperature, pulse and respiration rates are all raised. The breathing is shallow, painful and often grunting (p. 45), and accessory muscles of respiration, such as the sternomastoids and the alae nasi, may be in use. A patch of herpes sometimes breaks out on the lip or cheek and completes a characteristic clinical picture. There is cough which is usually dry at first but after a few days becomes productive of small quantities of mucoid sputum tinged with a typical rusty colour; frank haemoptysis is much less common. Pneumococci can be cultured from the sputum, and the white blood count is raised.

Before the days of antibiotics severe illness and high continuous fever persisted until sometime in the second week, when the temperature quickly fell and the patient within a few hours felt very much better. This event was known as the crisis. Nowadays the crisis is never seen, since within 48 hours of starting treatment with a suitable antibiotic the fever and accompanying constitutional symptoms have gone. At this stage, however, physical signs in the chest can still be detected and resolution of the inflammatory consolidation in the lung is not complete for another week or two.

Treatment Lobar pneumonia nearly always responds to injections of benzylpenicillin 500 000 units 6-hourly, which should be started without waiting for the result of the sputum culture. If clinical response is satisfactory treatment may be changed to oral penicillin (e.g. phenoxymethyl penicillin 250 mg 6-hourly). If the patient appears gravely ill it may be better to give ampicillin instead of penicillin; this is effective against a wider range of organisms, including *H. influenzae* which is often responsible for the pneumonic episodes in patients with chronic bronchitis. Patients allergic to the penicillins may be treated with tetracycline 250–500 mg 6-hourly or Septrin tab. two twice daily. Staphylococci may be resistant to penicillin, ampicillin and tetracycline and if this organism is suspected on clinical grounds it may be better to start treatment with a combination of cloxacillin and erythromycin. Treatment should be reviewed when the result of the sputum culture comes through, but it should be noted that the clinical effect of the drug being given is a piece of evidence just as important as the sensitivity test done in the laboratory in helping the physician to decide on further treatment.

Severe pleuritic pain is best treated with intramuscular pethidine 100 mg or subcutaneous morphine 15 mg. Persistent unproductive cough may be relieved by linctus pholcodine co. 4–8 ml. If the patient becomes cyanosed oxygen must be given, but the oxygen tent or mask may frighten or distress the patient and careful reassurance and encouragement are important.

Nursing Care With the use of the appropriate antibiotic complications are rare, but good nursing care is of primary importance.

The patient requires plenty of fresh air, but protection from draughts. The painful shallow breathing is relieved by nursing the patient sitting up, but the pillows must be adjusted for the comfort of each particular patient. A support for the feet is useful in preventing the patient slipping down the bed. Bedclothes must be light and warm, and a gown opening down the front is the most practical, as it minimises the amount of movement when the chest has to be examined. Rest is all important and there should not be disturbance for treatments and examinations. The patient should do very little for himself. He should have help with eating, drinking and expectorating; paper handkerchiefs are required to deal with tenacious sputum coughed up in the early stages. Daily bathing is necessary and beneficial, but the nurse must remember it can be exhausting and may have to be modified. All nursing care must be carried out with the greatest expediency; two nurses are required for turning the patient, making the bed and lifting him on and off bedpans.

Because of the toxaemia and tendency to breathe through the mouth, the tongue is coated and dry, and the lips tend to crack. Regular treatment of the mouth is necessary, and petroleum jelly should be applied to the lips. The patches of herpes which occur are best treated by dabbing with methylated spirit or an antiseptic powder.

The temperature, pulse, and respiration are taken and recorded 4-hourly; the temperature may have to be taken in the axilla or per rectum if there is severe dyspnoea. Persistent hyperpyrexia may necessitate tepid sponging. An accurate estimation of the respiration rate is essential, and any change in volume or regularity of the pulse must be reported, as it may be an indication of heart failure.

The importance of rest and avoidance of unnecessary disturbance have been emphasised, but changing the patient's position when nursing care and treatments are carried out is important in the prevention of hypostatic effects and pressure sores.

As in any febrile illness, the urinary output will be scanty at first, but with adequate fluid intake is soon adjusted. The urine should be tested for the presence of albumin. Abdominal distension may be troublesome and adds to respiratory distress; it can be relieved by passing a flatus tube. Glycerine suppositories or mild aperients such as isogel may be necessary to stimulate bowel action.

If pain of the pleuritic type is distressing, application of heat in the form of an electric pad may give relief. Alternatively a kaolin poultice can be used, but care must be taken that the patient lies on the poultice instead of the heavy poultice lying on his chest, and the bandage must not interfere with respiratory movement. If pain is very severe, pethidine 100 mg or morphine 20 mg may be ordered. The beneficial effect of these drugs in promoting rest outweighs the danger of respiratory depression. If cyanosis is severe, inhalations of oxygen will be necessary. This may entail placing the patient in an oxygen tent or using a Venti-mask, and as either method may distress him, careful explanation and reassurance are important.

During the early stage the cough is unproductive and very exhausting; a warm drink will often relieve it, and a depressant mixture such as linctus codeine 5–10 ml may be given. Later the cough will be productive and expectoration is encouraged. Every effort must be made to induce sleep; cool sponging or bathing of the hands and face will help to make the patient comfortable before hypnotic or analgesic drugs are given. Delirium may come on at night, and all measures must be taken to prevent this serious complication.

In the acute stage 3 litres of fluid must be given in the 24 hours, but as dyspnoea may make drinking difficult, small amounts only should be given at a time. The nurse will encourage the patient by varying the drinks. Bovril and Marmite are valuable when there has been excessive sweating, and slices of fresh fruit are refreshing and help to keep the mouth clean. Gradually a light, nourishing diet will be given, and during convalescence his diet should be normal, but with added protein.

The length of time the patient has to remain in bed depends on his age and the severity of the illness. Generally speaking he will be allowed up a couple of days after the temperature is normal. Breathing exercises should be commenced when the temperature falls and should be continued throughout convalescence, the length of which depends on the occupation and environment to which he has to return.

Complications

1 **Delayed Resolution** The time taken for the lung to return to its normal healthy state and for the X-ray to become clear varies a good deal in different patients. If there are residual clinical or radiological signs after about a month, it is very important to investigate the possibility that the pneumonia may not have been a primary infection but secondary to an underlying disease such as bronchial carcinoma, bronchiectasis or tuberculosis. The appropriate investigations are indicated in the sections on these diseases.

2 **Empyema** This is a collection of pus in the pleural cavity, and it should be suspected during the course of pneumonia or after apparent clinical recovery from pneumonia if the patient develops a swinging fever, high in the evening and down to normal or near normal in the morning. Severe constitutional symptoms, malaise, anorexia and heavy sweats are also likely to be present. The white blood count is very high, physical signs of fluid in the pleural cavity are found and the diagnosis is established by withdrawing pus through a wide-bore needle inserted into the chest in the area where the signs have been found. If the pus is thin, daily aspirations and installation of penicillin 500 000 units into the pleural cavity, together with a course of systemic penicillin injections, may be tried; but in many patients the pus is too thick to be removed satisfactorily in this way and surgical drainage of the empyema is necessary.

Broncho-pneumonia

Broncho-pneumonia is a complication of acute bronchitis and is seen most commonly in the very young and very old. In children it occurs with the acute specific fevers, particularly measles and whooping cough; in adults it results from respiratory infections such as influenza in patients weakened by other diseases or by old age, or from an acute exacerbation in a long-standing chronic bronchitis.

Acute bronchitis is described on p. 49. The transition from acute bronchitis to broncho-pneumonia is marked by the patient becoming more gravely ill, with further increase in the temperature, pulse and respiratory rates, and usually the onset of cyanosis. In contrast to lobar pneumonia, the physical signs are not confined to one lobe, but are generalised over both lungs, and the fever, instead of being continuous, tends to be swinging in type. There is always severe cough and usually profuse purulent sputum, which may occasionally be bloodstained.

Treatment Broncho-pneumonia is treated along the same lines as lobar pneumonia, but the clinical response is usually slower. Frequently treatment of the broncho-pneumonia is simply an episode in the management of the chronic bronchitis or bronchiectasis which underlies it.

Legionnaires' Disease

This unusual type of pneumonia occurs sporadically and is due to the organism *Legionella pneumophila.* General constitutional symptoms such as fever, malaise, rigors, headache, muscle pains, vomiting and mental confusion may be more prominent than cough and pleuritic pain but the chest X-ray shows segmental or lobar consolidation, which may be widespread and slow to clear. Clinical severity varies from a mild pneumonia to a rapidly fatal illness. **Diagnosis** depends on isolation of the organism from sputum and **treatment** is with erythromycin in full doses.

Bronchiectasis

The essential pathological change in bronchiectasis is dilatation of the bronchi in the diseased part of the lung. This dilatation may come about in a number of different ways. In many patients the trouble starts with an attack of broncho-pneumonia complicating one of the childhood fevers, particularly whooping cough or measles, and the first event is blocking of some of the smaller bronchi by plugs of sticky mucus. When the air in the alveoli supplied by these bronchi has been absorbed into the blood, no more air can get into them, so that they collapse like empty balloons, and the bronchi proximal to the obstruction dilate to take up the space in the chest which the air-filled alveoli previously occupied. At this stage permanent bronchiectasis can be prevented if the obstructing plugs of mucus are removed, as they nearly always can be, by vigorous physiotherapy: that is, by firm percussion on the chest wall to loosen the mucus and breathing exercises and postural coughing to encourage its expulsion. If this is achieved the alveoli re-expand and the bronchi return to their normal size. If the obstruction is allowed to persist, however, the affected bronchi remain in their dilated position and permanent bronchiectasis results. Destruction of the elastic tissue in the wall of the bronchi by the original infection may be another factor causing the dilatation.

In another group of patients the sequence of events starts with complete obstruction of the main bronchus to a lobe, usually the right middle lobe, by an enlarged tuberculous lymph-node at the hilum of the lung. This causes absorption collapse of all the alveoli in the lobe in the way described above. By the time the lymph-node has shrunk sufficiently to allow air into the bronchus again, many of the collapsed alveoli have become 'stuck' and fail to re-expand, so that compensatory dilatation of the bronchi occurs to take up the space they previously filled.

The distortion of the bronchi and impaired function of the affected segments of lung interfere with the normal movement of the film of mucus which covers the bronchial mucous membranes (p. 42). In consequence pools of mucus collect in the dilated bronchi and sooner or later they become infected. Chronic inflammatory changes now develop in the affected bronchi, and in the winter a respiratory infection may cause this inflammation to flare up and spread to the lung surrounding the bronchi, causing broncho-pneumonia. Broncho-pneumonia tends to cause scarring of the lung, so that each attack causes further damage, and eventually there may be extensive fibrosis of the affected lobe or lobes of the lung.

Clinical Features The main symptom is chronic cough productive of large quantities of purulent sputum (see p. 43). Coughing of blood (haemoptysis) is also quite common, and according to the extent of the disease in the lungs there may be mild or severe shortness of breath. Exacerbations of the disease in the winter cause increase in the symptoms, with fever and general malaise. The breath is sometimes very offensive and many patients develop clubbing of the fingers, which is therefore an important physical sign.

The commonest complication is broncho-pneumonia (p. 51). Much rarer, but very serious when they occur, are empyema (p. 55) and abscess in the brain. The latter develops when a portion of infected blood-clot from the diseased part of the lung becomes detached, passes along the pulmonary vein to the left side of the heart and is then swept up the carotid artery to become impacted in a small vessel in the brain.

Treatment

(*a*) **Medical** It must be remembered that patients who have bronchiectasis are often very sensitive and tend to withdraw from social contacts because of the persistent cough and sputum, which is unpleasant for patient and friends alike. Many of the victims of this disease are children. They are often considered backward and dull, but this is usually due to the school hours they have missed rather than lack of ability. Adults and children alike require understanding and sympathy and will quickly respond to the nurse who does not appear to be repulsed by their symptoms. The symptoms can nearly always be satisfactorily controlled and the complications largely prevented by regular and competent postural drainage. The patient is taught the position in which secretions which have collected in the dilated bronchi will flow under gravity towards the main bronchi and trachea, whence they can be expelled by coughing.

In the majority of patients who have bronchiectasis the lower lobes are affected. Postural drainage is achieved by leaning face downwards over the side of the bed with the hands on the floor. Alternatively the bed is raised 30 cm, the patient lying on his face or side, according to the part of the lobe affected. Postural drainage of the right middle lobe is achieved by placing the patient on his back with a pillow under the right side of the chest and the foot of the bed slightly raised. When the upper lobe is affected, drainage will take place if the patient is sitting up, leaning towards the unaffected side. The appropriate position must be adopted for at least 10 minutes twice a day, and forcible coughing should be continued until no more sputum will come up. Drainage of the secretions can often be improved by 'clapping' on the chest over the affected bronchi. The physiotherapist or the nurse may carry out this procedure, but later the patient's relatives will have to be instructed. Postural drainage should be carried out first thing in the morning, before the patient gets up. At this time of the day there will be a large quantity of sputum which has collected during the night. It may be necessary to repeat this treatment before the mid-day and evening meal. A hot drink given before each treatment will increase expectoration.

The amount of sputum must be measured and recorded daily, and to facilitate this sputum mugs should be graded in fluid ml. A measured amount of plain water or, if preferred, a colourless antiseptic lotion should be put in the mug to prevent the sputum from adhering. The clean mug must be brought to the patient before the used one is removed; on no account must the patient be left without a sputum mug. Postural drainage must of course be practised regularly throughout the whole of the patient's life.

Fluids and Diet The patient's appetite will be poor because he finds coughing aggravated by eating. He also has an unpleasant taste in his mouth due to the copious and often foul-smelling sputum coughed up. It is essential to improve his general condition, and every effort must be made to stimulate his appetite. Plenty of fluid must be given, food must be tempting and given in small quantities. A well-balanced diet is essential and extra protein for tissue repair can be introduced by giving casilan or complan and milk-drinks between meals. Additional ascorbic acid and vitamin B are also necessary.

When the patient first comes into hospital it may be necessary for him to eat his meals by his bed. As soon as the cough and sputum have been reasonably controlled he should be encouraged to join the other patients at the table.

General exercise is beneficial, and during most of the time investigations and treatments are being carried out the patient is up and about. Oral hygiene is of particular importance. Frequent mouth-washes will be necessary, and the patient should clean his teeth before all meals.

While the patient is in hospital the medical social worker investigates living conditions, and if these are not satisfactory the doctor will communicate with the local authorities in order to procure a more suitable environment. Damp, ill-ventilated houses and overcrowding are detrimental, and the patient may not be able to carry out his own treatment satisfactorily. The patient himself must take every possible care to avoid colds and other respiratory infections.

Antibiotics have little place in the treatment of bronchiectasis, but a course of penicillin or tetracycline may be given when an acute febrile exacerbation occurs.

(*b*) **Surgical** What amounts to complete cure of bronchiectasis can be achieved only by removal of the diseased part of the lung, but unfortunately very few bronchiectatics are suitable for this operation. The ideal patient for surgical treatment is the child or young adult with severe bronchiectasis completely confined to one lobe. Usually, however, when the disease affects only one lobe the symptoms can be controlled so well by simple medical measures that the risk of lobectomy is hardly justified; and when the symptoms are more severe the disease is so widespread in both lungs that too little healthy lung would be left if it were extirpated. Before deciding about operation it is essential, therefore, to know the full extent of the disease in both lungs. This is demonstrated by bronchography: that is, by injecting radio-opaque fluid into the larynx, positioning the patient so that the bronchi of each of the five lobes are filled in turn and then taking a chest X-ray.

Spontaneous Pneumothorax

Any pulmonary lesion which ruptures through the surface of the lung and its covering layer of visceral pleura allows air at atmospheric pressure to flow from the bronchi into the pleural space and the lung collapses. This is a spontaneous pneumothorax. The common cause is rupture of a small congenital subpleural vesicle in otherwise healthy young adults. The patient usually complains of sudden pain and shortness of breath; examination of the chest reveals weak or absent breath sounds on the affected side; and the chest X-ray is diagnostic. In most patients the hole in the pleura heals in a few days, the air in the pleural cavity is absorbed and the lung re-expands without specific treatment, but when the opening into the pleural cavity acts as a one-way valve the movements of respiration pump air into the pleural cavity under increasing pressure. This is a tension pneumothorax and is a medical emergency; a needle, preferably connected by tubing to an under-water seal, must be inserted into the chest to let the air out. Any large or persistent pneumothorax may need to be treated in this way.

Asthma

Patients with bronchial asthma suffer attacks of wheezing and difficulty in breathing due either to bronchial spasm or to partial obstruction of the bronchi by sticky secretions, or more commonly to a combination of both these factors. The cause of the disease is complex, and in most patients several of the following influences contribute to its development.

1 **Heredity** Particularly when the asthma starts in childhood or adolescence, there is likely to be a positive family history, either of asthma itself or of some other allergic disorder such as hay fever or urticaria. Migraine in the mother or father is a common finding.

2 **Allergy** An allergic person is one who has become abnormally sensitive to some substance with which he comes into contact; in the allergic asthmatic, for example, exposure to the substance in question causes contraction of the bronchial muscles and exudation

into the bronchi of sticky mucus, or in other words it brings on an attack of asthma. There are a large number of substances to which the asthmatic may become allergic, and they fall into two main groups: those which are in the atmosphere and are inhaled by the patient, and those in the food which are ingested by the patient. Of these two groups the inhalants are much the more important: common examples are pollen and spores from plants, moulds, mites in house dust, animal hair, dandruff and face-powder. Foodstuffs are much less often to blame, but among those which may induce attacks are eggs, milk, fish—particularly shell-fish—certain fruits and chocolate.

The patient's history is the best guide to whether allergy plays an important part in his asthma. Thus, if the attacks occur only in the spring and early summer it is reasonable to suspect that pollens are responsible, or it may be found that attacks are induced by eating some particular food or by going into a room containing a cat or a dog. Skin tests can also be done. A drop of a specially prepared solution of the substance suspected is placed on the skin and a superficial scratch made through it, and if the result is positive a raised weal appears at the site of the scratch within 10 or 15 minutes. In practice, however, skin testing is much less helpful than a carefully taken history in the investigation and treatment of asthma.

3 Infection Infections in either the upper or lower respiratory tract are often important factors. In asthmatic children, in whom allergy is usually also much in evidence, colds in the head are often followed by attacks of wheezing; allergy is usually much less prominent when asthma starts later in life, and in this group of patients the asthma often appears as a complication of chronic bronchitis.

4 Reflex factors The bronchi are supplied by the vagus nerve, and in many asthmatics various stimuli may induce attacks by a reflex mechanism. Common examples are exertion, sudden exposure to cold air, distension of the stomach by a heavy meal and constipation.

5 Psychological influences play some part in nearly every asthmatic and quite often they appear to be mainly responsible, if not in starting the asthma, at least in maintaining it. Anxieties and worries of various kinds, a sense of frustration or very frequently discord and an atmosphere of tension in the home, are often found underlying the tension in the bronchi; and unless these influences are appreciated and the patient handled with sympathetic understanding, tact and firmness, and unless everything possible is done to ease the difficulties in his life, the response to treatment is not likely to be very satisfactory.

Clinical Features An attack of asthma usually comes on fairly suddenly and lasts about an hour or so, but the duration varies a good deal; many asthmatics have bad spells lasting some weeks, and during these periods they may be continuously rather wheezy and suffer frequent acute exacerbations, especially during the night. When a severe attack lasts more than a day or so the patient is said to be in status asthmaticus. During the attack the patient complains of tightness in the chest and has great difficulty in breathing, particularly in the expiratory phase of respiration (see p. 45). There is often cough, which is dry at first, but towards the end of the attack produces some rather sticky, tight little pellets of mucoid sputum. The sputum is purulent only when there is associated infection in the respiratory tract.

Between attacks the structure and function of the lungs return to normal except in those patients with long-standing severe asthma, who develop the complication known as emphysema. As a result of frequent severe over-distension the lungs lose their elasticity and remain permanently expanded; their function is correspondingly impaired, and the patient is short of breath even when not in an attack of asthma.

Treatment: (*a*) **During attacks** An attack can usually be stopped if the patient uses a pressurised aerosol containing Salbutamol (Ventolin inhaler), particularly if he does so at the onset of symptoms. Salbutamol has a more prolonged action than isoprenaline and does not cause cardiovascular side-effects such as palpitations. Salbutamol is therefore the safer drug to take in this way; it is thought that the increased mortality from asthma in childhood which occurred in this country in the 1950s and 1960s was due to overuse of pressurised aerosols containing isoprenaline. Alternatively the patient may be given aminophylline 0.25–0.5 g in 10–20 ml sterile water by slow intravenous injection.

Severe status asthmaticus which has not responded to the above drugs is a dangerous illness which is not infrequently fatal. Although the patient is exhausted by sleeplessness and the enormous effort expended in breathing, on no account must he be given morphine or any other derivative of opium, since the resulting depression of respiration would almost certainly kill him. Indeed, it is best to avoid giving any sedative, but if it is felt that restlessness is increasing the exhaustion to a dangerous extent, diazepam (Valium) 2–5 mg may be given with advantage at bedtime. Steroids may be life-saving. Prednisolone is given, 50 mg on the first day, 30 mg on the second day and 20 mg daily thereafter. A more rapid response may be obtained by giving IV hydrocortisone 200 mg 3-hourly and when the patient is gravely ill this is usually given in an intravenous infusion which also corrects the dehydration. Improvement usually occurs within a day or so and the steroid should then be tailed off.

(*b*) **Treatment between attacks** has to be planned individually for each patient, and before this can be done intelligently a careful assessment must be made of the various possible causative factors indicated above. The aim of treatment is to prevent attacks, for the longer the patient can be kept free of asthma the less likely is it to return; or, as one famous physician put it, 'the way to treat asthma is not to get it'.

The psychological handling of the patient is of the utmost importance. The nurse must be a good and sympathetic listener, so that the asthmatic can get his various worries and troubles literally 'off his chest'; at the same time there must be no unnecessary fussing over his symptoms and an atmosphere of calm confidence must be preserved at all times.

With regard to the allergic factor, it is nearly always advisable for the asthmatic to avoid contact as far as possible with the various substances to which he is or may become sensitive: his bedroom should therefore be bare and spartan, containing no cushions, curtains or other soft furnishings which harbour dust; feather quilts should be avoided; and preferably in place of feather pillows and hair mattress sorbo rubber substitutes should be used. When there is a clear-cut allergy—for example, to pollen—specific desensitisation may be attempted. This is done by giving injections of a solution of the substance in question about once a week, starting with a very small dose and gradually increasing it until the patient has a slight reaction. At the next injection the dose is reduced slightly, and then steadily increased again over the next week or two until another reaction occurs, when the procedure is repeated. In this way the patient gradually comes to tolerate quite a large dose, or in other words he becomes desensitised. Two warnings must be heeded by anyone giving these desensitising injections. Firstly, a syringe charged with 1/1000 adrenaline must always be kept ready and an injection of 0.5 ml with 10 mg of chlorpheniramine given at once if the patient develops any local reaction, such as irritation at the site of the injection, or general reaction, such as wheezing or faintness. The patient must also be kept under observation for at least half-an-hour after each injection is given. Secondly, desensitisation against pollens must be completed before the end of April, as severe and even fatal reactions may occur if injections are given when pollens are actually present in the atmosphere.

Disodium cromoglycate (Intal), inhaled 3 or 4 times daily using a device known as a spinhaler, has proved very helpful in reducing the frequency and severity of attacks in which the allergic factor appears to be prominent.

With regard to the reflex induction of attacks, patients should be warned to avoid large, heavy meals, particularly in the evening, and constipation should be corrected. In addition, the patient's history frequently reveals other ways in which attention to healthy habits of living will help to cut down the number and severity of his attacks.

For the prevention of attacks regular administration of salbutamol tablets, 2 mg four times daily, is often helpful but occasionally causes troublesome shakiness. An aminophylline suppository at bedtime may be very effective in preventing nocturnal attacks.

Finally, all asthmatics should be taught special breathing exercises and should carry them out regularly for the rest of their lives. These exercises are particularly designed to encourage the use of the diaphragm in inspiration and the use of the abdominal muscles in increasing the force of expiration; they are of benefit to the asthmatic not only in helping him to overcome the obstruction to breathing during the attacks, but also in preventing or reducing the incidence of emphysema.

A small group of patients have very severe chronic asthma which can be controlled only by continuous steroid therapy. Initial dosage of 30–40 mg prednisolone is gradually reduced to the minimum effective level, which preferably should not be higher than 10 mg daily. A beclomethasone (Becotide) inhaler enables a steroid to be given without danger of systemic side-effects.

Carcinoma of the Bronchus

This disease has become much more common in recent years. It occurs in middle age, particularly between the ages 40 and 60, and affects men several times more often than women. The cause is unknown, but it has been shown that the risk of acquiring it is much greater in heavy cigarette-smokers and in those who live in the polluted atmosphere of industrial areas.

The tumour usually develops in one of the main bronchi, and by pressing on neighbouring healthy epithelium it tends to elicit the cough reflex. Cough is therefore the commonest early symptom and is dry at first; but later erosion of blood vessels by the tumour, or infection developing beyond it, cause bloodstained or mucopurulent sputum to appear. As the carcinoma increases in size the bronchus in which it is growing becomes increasingly obstructed, so that the corresponding segment or lobe of the lung loses its air supply and collapses like an empty balloon. The patient now notices some shortness of breath. A persistent wheeze over the site of the bronchial obstruction and a dull, deep-seated pain in the chest are other common symptoms. It is usually not until the later stages of the disease that general weakness, loss of weight, anaemia and clubbing of the fingers make their appearance, and it is important that the diagnosis should be made earlier than this if the patient is to have a chance of cure.

The possibility of this disease should be considered, therefore, in every middle-aged patient who has not previously had any respiratory trouble and who develops persistent symptoms such as those mentioned above. Clinical or radiological examination of the chest may then show evidence of absorption collapse in the affected lobe of the lung, and the diagnosis is finally established by bronchoscopy. The bronchoscope is passed down into the trachea either with the patient under general anaesthesia or after locally anaesthetising the throat and larynx, and through the instrument the growth can be seen and a small portion of it removed for examination.

Complications Spread of the cancer cells may lead to the development of secondary growths (metastases) in various parts of the body. Local spread within the chest leads to involvement of the mediastinal lymph-nodes and the pleura, and a bloodstained pleural effusion often results. When the cancer cells get into the bloodstream they may be carried to any part of the body: the commonest places where metastases actually grow are bones such as the vertebrae and ribs, where they cause severe backache or pain in the chest; the skin, where they appear as hard fixed lumps; the liver, which consequently enlarges and becomes irregular; and the brain, where they cause the symptoms and signs of brain tumours.

Another important complication is infection in the segment of lung whose bronchus has been obstructed by the carcinoma.

Patients quite often do not seek medical advice until this has occurred, and there is a danger that they may be treated for pneumonia or lung abscess without the underlying cause being recognised. The possibility of bronchial carcinoma should therefore be suspected in any middle-aged patient whose 'pneumonia' does not respond quickly and completely to the treatment given.

Treatment The only hope of cure lies in surgical removal of the affected lung (pneumonectomy) or lobe (lobectomy). Unfortunately many patients cannot be treated in this way, either because they are not fit enough to withstand the operation or because the carcinoma has already metastasised, and of those who do undergo operation only some 20 per cent survive for 5 years or longer. The results of treatment are therefore among the worst for cancer in any part of the body.

Radiotherapy is often helpful in relieving distressing symptoms such as suffocating dyspnoea, but probably does not prolong life. The average length of survival of patients unsuitable for surgery is about 9 months.

Tuberculosis

While the annual death rate from carcinoma of the bronchus has been increasing in recent years, there has been a corresponding fall in the mortality from tuberculosis. There are, however, no grounds for complacency with regard to the latter disease, which still causes serious and prolonged ill-health in large numbers of young adults at the time of life when illness has the most serious economic and social consequences. Furthermore, being due to infection with the tubercle bacillus, whose methods of dissemination are well known, tuberculosis is essentially a preventible disease whose continued existence in the community presents a challenge to all workers in the field of public health and social medicine.

Infection and Immunity There are two main types of tubercle bacilli: the bovine and the human. The former cause tuberculosis in cattle, but when they spread to human beings in milk from infected cows they give rise to human tuberculosis indistinguishable from that due to 'human' bacilli, which spread directly from one human patient to another. At the present time in England and Wales about 10 per cent and in Scotland about 20 per cent of tuberculous patients are infected with 'bovine' bacilli.

In order to cause tuberculosis, tubercle bacilli must first gain access to the patient and then overcome his defences or immunity. Access to potential victims is usually achieved by so-called 'droplet infection': patients with open phthisis (that is, those who have tubercle bacilli in their sputum) spray large numbers of bacilli into the surrounding atmosphere in coughing, sneezing and talking, and anyone else in the same room is likely to inhale them into his lungs. Alternatively but less commonly the bacilli may be transmitted to the patient in infected milk. What happens next depends partly on the number of bacilli reaching the patient and partly on his state of immunity; in other words, even good defences against tuberculosis may be overcome if the individual is in close and prolonged contact with open phthisis and receives an overwhelming dose of tubercle bacilli.

Immunity is of two types: 'natural' and 'acquired'. **Natural immunity** is the inherited resistance of the body against tuberculosis, and it varies a good deal in different people; the Irish, for example, appear generally speaking to have less natural immunity than the English and are consequently more susceptible to tuberculosis. **Acquired immunity** is the additional resistance to infection a patient achieves when he has overcome and recovered from his primary tuberculous infection.

In this country up to 1950 over 95% of urban dwellers unknowingly had their first (or 'primary') tuberculous infection before reaching adult life and a small number still do so. The site of this infection is either the lung, the tonsillar area or the lower ileum; a very small local lesion results, and the tubercle bacilli pass on to cause great enlargement of the regional lymph-nodes either in the mediastinum, the neck or the mesentery, according to the site of infection. Usually the defences of the body prevent the bacilli spreading further than the regional lymph-nodes, and healing of the lesions takes place, in the course of which calcification of the nodes occurs and remains as a permanent record of the battle. Sometimes, however, the lesions do not heal completely, but remain quiescent until perhaps months or even years later, when they may liberate some tubercle bacilli into the bloodstream, by which they are transported to cause tuberculosis in another part of the body, such as the kidney or epididymus, a bone or a joint. In another small group of patients the primary infection overwhelms the natural defences and tubercle bacilli are carried in the blood to every organ of the body, where they form numerous lesions known as miliary tubercles. This type of disease is therefore called miliary tuberculosis. Involvement of the central nervous system by this process often leads to tuberculous meningitis, and until a few years ago death was the almost invariable outcome. Nowadays, fortunately, if the diagnosis of miliary tuberculosis is made early enough and vigorous treatment instituted with antituberculous drugs, many of these patients can be restored to good health.

As already mentioned, in the vast majority of people the primary tuberculous infection heals without ever causing symptoms. The fact that this has occurred can be demonstrated by a tuberculin test such as the Mantoux, which is performed in the following way. 0.1 ml of a 1/10 000 dilution of old tuberculin (which is an extract of dead tubercle bacilli) is injected intradermally (that is, into the skin) of the forearm, and if the patient has never had any tuberculous lesion no local reaction occurs. The test must then be repeated with stronger solutions of tuberculin—1/1000 and if necessary 1/100—before the patient is regarded as Mantoux negative. The primary infection with tuberculosis not only leaves the patient with acquired immunity, it also leaves his tissues permanently sensitised (or allergic) to tuberculin, so that when he is Mantoux tested the site of the injection becomes red and swollen. The Mantoux reaction is regarded as positive when there is a raised area at least 5 mm in diameter surrounded by a red flush when the arm is examined 48 hours after the injection.

It will be clear from the above discussion that people who are Mantoux positive have an acquired as well as a natural immunity against tuberculosis, whereas those who are Mantoux negative have only their natural immunity. In other words, the latter run a greater risk of contracting tuberculosis if exposed to infection. For this reason nurses, medical students and others who come into contact with tuberculous patients are given Mantoux tests and an attempt is made to convert those who are Mantoux negative to Mantoux positive by BCG vaccination. This involves inoculation into the skin of the arm or leg of a special culture of tubercle bacilli which have been treated in such a way that they can no longer cause tuberculosis, though they can still stimulate the body's defences and promote acquired immunity in the same way as the primary tuberculous infection.

'Postprimary' Tuberculosis

People who have recovered from their primary tuberculous infection, and who possess therefore both natural and acquired immunity, may nevertheless develop 'postprimary' tuberculosis if their immunity is reduced by some debilitating process such as undernourishment, overwork, chronic alcoholism or diabetes, or if they live or work in close contact with someone suffering from open phthisis and are bombarded with enormous numbers of tubercle bacilli. Frequently it is a combination of both these factors that allows the disease to gain a foothold. As the patient's tissues are allergic to tuberculin as a result of the primary infection, the tubercle bacilli this time do not pass through to the regional lymphatic nodes, but are caught up in the large reaction which occurs at the site of infection in the subapical portion of one of the two upper lobes of the lungs. A long struggle now takes place between the tubercle bacilli, which try to spread the disease throughout the lungs, and the body's defences, which try to localise it by laying down fibrous tissue to wall it off; and the course of the disease is very variable according to the degree of success achieved by either side. The centre of the lesion tends to undergo a characteristic type of necrosis known as caseation (so called because the dead tissue is converted into a cheese-like substance), and the tuberculous cavity results when this necrotic material erodes into a bronchus and is coughed up. This type of disease is known as fibrocaseous pulmonary tuberculosis, and it is the common variety found in young adults.

Symptoms Early diagnosis is extremely important if the patient is to have the best chance of recovery, so that one must not wait until signs of grave ill-health have appeared before thinking of tuberculosis. There are a number of ways in which the disease may come to light clinically:

1 **Haemoptysis.** Sometimes the first symptom is the coughing up of a mouthful of bright-red blood; and when a young adult who has had no previous respiratory trouble has a haemoptysis of this order the possibility of tuberculosis must be investigated without delay.

2 **Chronic productive cough.** The characteristics of tuberculous sputum are indicated on p. 44. Anyone may cough up a little mucoid sputum for a week or so after a cold, but when the cough is more persistent, and particularly if there are also constitutional symptoms as outlined below, the chest should be X-rayed and the sputum examined for tubercle bacilli.

3 **Constitutional symptoms.** These are the general effects on the body of the tuberculosis in the lungs, and include tiredness, loss of weight, indigestion, evening fever, night sweats and amenorrhoea.

4 **Pleurisy with effusion.** Aspiration of the chest reveals a clear, straw-coloured fluid which is sterile on culture, and its tuberculous nature can sometimes be proved by inoculating it into a guinea-pig. The effusion is probably an allergic response of the pleura to an underlying tuberculous lesion, and as about 25 per cent of these patients develop frank pulmonary tuberculosis within the next 5 years, they must all be kept under observation and have periodic chest X-rays during this period.

5 **Erythema nodosum** is a condition in which bluish-red, slightly raised lesions about an inch in diameter appear on the front of the legs, and is sometimes an allergic response to tuberculosis elsewhere in the body.

6 Finally, pulmonary tuberculosis is now sometimes detected before any symptoms have appeared by means of routine *mass miniature radiography*.

Diagnosis X-ray of the chest reveals characteristic shadows, particularly in the upper lobes, but sometimes it is difficult to decide whether these shadows represent active or healed lesions. Frequently the other clinical findings supply the answer to this question: for example, if the patient has cough, fever, a raised sedimentation rate (normal up to 10 mm in 1 hour) and tubercle bacilli in his sputum there is of course no doubt that his disease is active. If he is quite well clinically, the significance of the shadows on the X-ray may not be decided until other films have been taken at intervals of a few weeks; if the shadows remain exactly the same in all of them, the lesions are probably inactive. Alternatively, special X-rays may be taken by what is called tomography. This is a technique which enables the focus of the X-rays to be adjusted to different depths in the chest so that pictures of a series of slices through the lungs can be obtained. By this means the lesions can be studied in greater detail, and if any cavitation is seen in the centre of them, the disease is unquestionably still active.

A prolonged search must always be made for tubercle bacilli in the sputum. Discovery of the organism is not only the most certain way of establishing the diagnosis, it also indicates that the patient is infective and that special precautions must be taken to prevent the spread of infection. When sputum is sent to the laboratory the nurse must make sure that a representative sample of mucoid sputum from the lung is chosen; left to himself, the patient will often simply spit a little saliva into the pot. Other patients swallow all their sputum and are unable to produce any for examination; the specimens must therefore be obtained by washing out the stomach first thing in the morning. The pathologist detects tubercle bacilli by staining them and then demonstrating that the stain cannot be removed by soaking them in acid (as it can from other organisms). A positive report often states, therefore, that 'acid-fast bacilli' (or AFB) are present in the sputum.

Treatment For active tuberculosis complete rest with plenty of fresh air and good food is the most important part of the treatment. A course of chemotherapy must also be given, usually starting with three of the available antituberculous drugs since if any one is given alone the tubercle bacilli tend to become resistant to its action. The original combination of drugs used was streptomycin, isoniazid (INAH) and para-aminosalicylic acid (PAS), but increasingly streptomycin is being replaced by ethambutol, which is less toxic (though very rarely it causes blindness from optic atrophy, so the visual acuity must be checked every 4 weeks while this drug is given); and rifampicin is being preferred to PAS, which causes unpleasant gastro-intestinal symptoms.

Chemotherapy must be continued for 1–2 years after all evidence of activity in the disease has gone.

Surgical resection of the affected segments or lobes of the lung is very occasionally needed for patients with cavities which persist in spite of adequate rest and chemotherapy, or for those infected with tubercle bacilli resistant to chemotherapy.

The duration of the active stage of treatment is very variable, but is nearly always at least several months. It must be continued until all clinical evidence of activity in the disease has gone, and the patient is then gradually allowed to resume a more normal life. The process of rehabilitation is best undertaken at a sanatorium, where the patient's progress through the various stages of convalescence is carefully watched and controlled. When he is finally allowed to go home he is transferred to the care of the local chest clinic where periodic medical examinations and X-rays are carried out and any further treatment or investigation which may be needed is arranged. This supervision will continue for the rest of the patient's life or until the chest physician is quite satisfied that the disease has finally healed.

Nursing Care Any long illness such as pulmonary tuberculosis necessitates a great deal of readjustment on the part of the patient, and all concerned must do their utmost to help him through the long period of inactivity and rehabilitation.

To the majority of patients the knowledge that they are suffering from tuberculosis comes as a great shock and will immediately conjure up fears and anxieties. The patient will ask himself many questions: Will he get better? Will he be able to return to work? Has he infected his family or friends? How is he going to be able to support a family?—and so on. It is important that the medical social worker visit him as soon as possible to give specific information about his salary, tuberculosis allowance, assistance with rent and other expenses. He will also be reassured by knowing that contacts will have X-ray examinations and follow-ups, and that protective measures such as BCG vaccination are being given in the case of children. Advice regarding his own adjustment and prognosis must come from someone on whom he can rely, preferably his own doctor.

There will, however, be times when he will be despondent, irritable and moody or alternatively highly excitable. Great patience and understanding of his behaviour pattern are necessary on the part of all those concerned with his well being—doctor, nurse, medical social worker and relatives. Because the nurse is more constantly with him, he will depend on her to help him over many stages of readjustment until he is finally able to return to his home and take his place in society.

Ideally such patients should be nursed in a sanatorium, where the surroundings are healthy and where there are facilities for the treatment of all types of tuberculosis.

In the acute stage the patient is nursed at rest, and is not allowed to wash himself. In addition to the daily blanket bath, sponging is necessary when night sweats are profuse. Particular attention is paid to pressure areas, as the patient may be grossly emaciated. The mouth must be kept fresh and clean, and may require treatment 4-hourly. The patient will be easily exhausted, so all nursing procedures must be carried out gently and quickly. Two nurses should be available for bedmaking and for lifting him on and off bedpans. Temperature, pulse and respiration will be taken 4-hourly; a rectal temperature gives the most accurate recording. Although the patient requires as much rest as possible, reading and listening to the wireless will be beneficial, as these give him other interests. Adjustable bookrests are useful in preventing extra exertion.

Tuberculosis is a disease where wasting may be an outstanding feature, therefore a light diet high in protein is essential to build up general resistance. Unfortunately the chemotherapy given may tend to cause nausea and vomiting, and so affect the appetite. Meals should therefore be temptingly served, there should be as much variety of food as possible and small helpings to prevent the patient refusing the whole meal. The protein content of the diet can be supplemented by milk fortified with casilan (protein 26 g to 30 ml). Plenty of fluids should also be given to reduce the toxaemia. Only in extreme instances is it necessary for the patient to be fed. He will eat more when feeding himself. Careful arrangement of the patient before each meal will reduce the effort entailed to a minimum. The patient should be weighed at weekly intervals.

If the cough is productive it should not be discouraged, but the patient sometimes develops a dry, ineffectual cough which can be harmful, and he should be taught to control it. Linctus codeine at night will help to suppress an irritating cough.

Haemoptysis may occur at any time during the disease. A severe haemoptysis will be very frightening for the patient, and calm reassurance on the part of the nurse is essential. He must be kept as quiet as possible and, unless dyspnoeic, placed in a recumbent position on the affected side to prevent blood from spilling over into the other lung, which would cause spread of infection. An injection of morphia 20 mg will be given to help to control bleeding and to allay anxiety.

A colourless mouth-wash should be given to take away the unpleasant taste of blood, and the nurse should constantly observe her patient's condition without undue disturbance; the pulse should be taken and recorded quarter-hourly. Following the haemoptysis a further period of complete rest will be necessary.

As a guide to the effectiveness of the treatment the physician will require a series of three to six early morning specimens of sputum to be sent to the laboratory at intervals throughout the course of the disease. As already mentioned, it may be necessary for *gastric washings* to be carried out. The patient should have nothing to eat or drink from the previous evening. The procedure entails passing a nasogastric (Ryle's) tube, injecting 30 ml of distilled water down the tube and withdrawing the gastric contents.

As the condition improves many patients will find the enforced period of rest irksome, while others tend to become apathetic. Occupational therapy may stimulate the interest until activities can be increased. A strict regime of gradually increased exercise and periods of rest is essential during the convalescent period. The patient begins to participate in social activities, but it is also important that group activities should not be overdone to the exclusion of independent thought and action.

Throughout the illness relatives and friends are encouraged to visit as often as possible, so that family relationships will not suffer.

During the patient's stay in hospital the medical social worker will have investigated home conditions and sought the help of the local authority if any changes are necessary.

Prevention of Spread of Infection Broadly speaking, patients suffering from pulmonary tuberculosis can be divided into two categories:

1 'Open' tuberculosis with positive sputum;
2 'Closed' tuberculosis with negative sputum.

(1) The first group of patients, where possible, should be nursed in a sanatorium. If they are in a general hospital on a balcony or in a private room, full barrier precautions should be observed, and destructible cartons used for sputum. (2) For this group it is only necessary for eating and washing utensils to be kept separate.

All patients must be instructed regarding the necessity for using paper handkerchiefs. After use these should be placed in a paper bag by the patient's bed, collected and burnt daily. The dangers of coughing and the added risk entailed by close contact with relatives—e.g. kissing—must also be emphasised. All nurses must wear a mask when dealing with patients and should wash their hands after attendance on any of these patients.

Respiratory Failure

Measurement of the oxygen and carbon dioxide tension in arterial blood is used to assess the efficiency of respiration. The normal partial pressures are:

Oxygen (PO_2): 12 kPa (range 9.3–14.6)
Carbon dioxide (PCO_2): 5.3 kPa (range 4.8–5.9)

The patient is said to be in *respiratory failure* when the oxygen (PO_2) falls below 8 kPa and the carbon dioxide (PCO_2) rises above 7.7 kPa.

Patients with chronic lung disease are especially prone to respiratory failure when an acute illness supervenes, e.g. acute respiratory infection, pulmonary collapse from bronchial obstruction, pneumothorax, weakness of respiratory muscles from neurological diseases such as poliomyelitis, or depression of the respiratory centre in the brain stem from anoxia or poisons. Such patients require nursing in an intensive care unit where assisted respiration by positive-pressure ventilation is available.

4
Intensive Care Nursing

Nursing patients who require intensive care is challenging, demanding and highly satisfying. It is a field of work where high standards of theoretical knowledge and practical competence accompanied by skilled interpersonal relationships with patients, relatives, colleagues, medical staff and staff from other disciplines are essential. Competence in this sphere of nursing should be acquired even if there is no intention to specialise in it; all nurses should know how to look after patients on life-support machines and should learn how to deal efficiently with medical emergencies.

The Patient

Whatever special care an acutely ill patient needs his basic nursing care is still of vital importance. General hygiene, care of pressure areas, care of eyes, mouth, bladder and bowels must not be neglected. Aseptic procedures must be performed correctly as the vulnerability of acutely ill patients to secondary infections is high. The patient may be conscious or unconscious, unable to talk if he is receiving assistance from positive-pressure ventilation, and usually very apprehensive about his condition and the many pieces of apparatus that surround him (see Figure on p. 76). The nurse must employ every communication skill available by touch, expression and voice to make the patient feel secure and cared for. Questions must be carefully phrased so that a simple answer or nod of the head is all that is required from the patient. Relatives are usually very anxious and often bewildered by all the apparatus. They should be made to feel welcome and useful even if it is only to hold the patient's hand. They should be informed in an honest and understandable way about the condition of the patient and care should be taken to assess how they are reacting to the situation. Doctors, nurses, physiotherapists and technicians have to work as a united team and written and verbal observations must be accurate and communicated quickly to other members of the team.

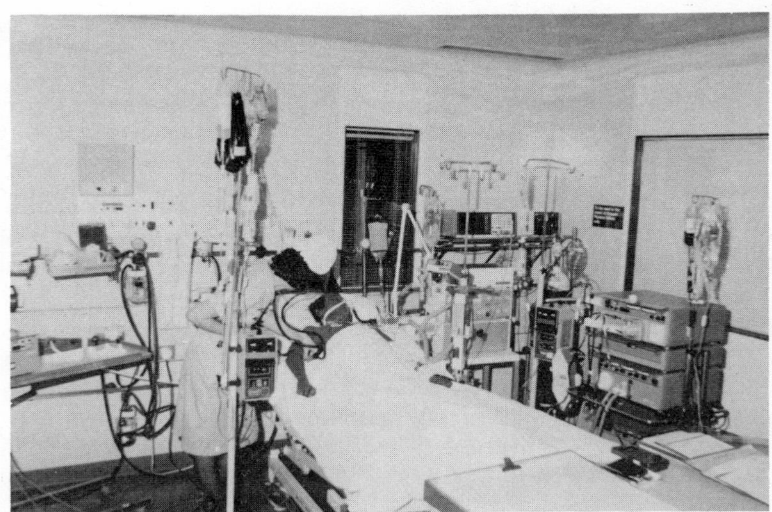

Patient with multiple systems failure requiring maximal support

Some of the equipment shown includes a teckmar infusion control pump, IVI stand holding intravenous feeding regime, CVP measurement equipment/fluid; *behind*, suction and intubation equipment; *on the table*, bed scales monitor.

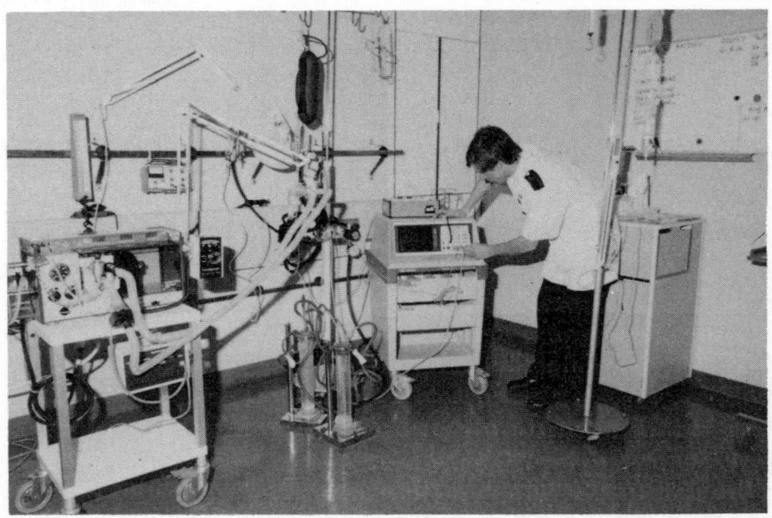

Typical room ready to receive back patient following cardiac surgery.

1. Ventilator, O_2 analyser, ventilator tubing/support; 2. Monitoring equipment (i.e. haemodynamic monitoring, ECG, temperature); 3. IV stand with CVP monitoring equipment; 4. IV stand with Fenwell bag for pressure monitoring attached to transducers behind; 5. Packing box with connections; 6. Manual BP manometer; 7. Drainage bottles attached to wall suction.

The Extended Role of the Qualified Nurse

Commonly nurses are taught and tested to ensure that they can administer intravenous drugs, but other procedures normally outside the role of the nurse may also be required of her. Each individual must ensure that she receives adequate tuition on each procedure and should undertake it only if she feels competent and is willing to assume the added responsibility. She must accept that if she makes a mistake she will be held accountable.

Nurses involved with patients requiring life support equipment or working in intensive care units are advised to consult specialist textbooks. It is strongly recommended that nurses working in these units should have undertaken the post registration course approved by the English National Board in order that they have sufficient knowledge to be safe and proficient in the care they give.

Bereavement

The mortality rate of patients requiring intensive care is inevitably high. Nurses must accept this and understand the needs of dying patients, their relatives, the other members of the care team and themselves. If a patient cannot be nursed back to health it is the nurse's duty to ensure that he dies with dignity, without pain and above all that he does not feel lonely. It requires both experience and sensitivity to be able to discuss this situation with patients and their relatives. Nurses must be able to deal appropriately and adequately with the patient who wishes to know that he is dying and equally so with the patient who does not. The nurse must also understand reactions such as aggression, fear, guilt, shock, mistrust and hysteria which some relatives may show. Above all she must have thought through her own reactions to the death of someone to whom she has devoted all her professional skill, care and emotional support for perhaps a long period of time. There are many excellent specialist texts now available on the subject of bereavement, and increasingly, special teams are being set up to advise on Terminal Care.

5

The Alimentary System

The Significance of Abdominal Pain

Pain is the commonest symptom of diseases affecting the abdominal organs, and certain of its characteristics are often helpful in diagnosis. The viscera are not sensitive structures: large tumours or other lesions in solid organs such as the liver, kidneys or spleen are quite painless; and if the stomach or intestine is exposed in a conscious patient it can be cut or burnt with diathermy, for example, without giving rise to any discomfort. How, then, is the pain of abdominal diseases produced? It arises in two main ways:

1 **Visceral Pain.** The only stimulus which causes pain in a hollow muscular organ, such as the stomach, duodenum and intestines, the bile ducts, the ureters or the uterus, is increased tension in its wall. Such increase in tension is usually due to spasm in the muscular wall or stretching from distension. The commonest example of this type of pain arises from strong peristaltic spasms in the colon induced by hard faecal masses resulting from constipation; and the word 'colic' has come to be used in a general sense for this type of pain, whether it arises in the colon or in any of the other muscular tubes mentioned above.

Colic has certain characteristic features which distinguish it from other types of abdominal pain. It comes in waves, working up to a crisis and then gradually subsiding again; when severe, it causes the patient to double up or even writhe about in agony; warmth to the abdomen helps to relieve it; reflex vomiting often accompanies it, particularly at the onset, and it is poorly localised, the patient indicating its situation with a wave of the hand rather than with a pointing finger. Furthermore, this type of pain is not always felt over the organ producing it, but is often 'referred' to an area of skin supplied from the same spinal segment as the organ in question. Thus, pain is felt in the mid-line of the epigastrium from lesions on the stomach or duodenum; small intestine colic is felt round the umbilicus; large intestine colic in the lower abdomen; biliary colic in the right upper quadrant of the abdomen; renal colic in the loin, often radiating round to the iliac fossa and down into the testicle on the same side; and uterine colic usually in the lower abdomen.

2 **Pain due to Inflammation of the Parietal Peritoneum,** on

the other hand, is a sharp, severe, steady pain accurately localised over the site of the inflammation, and since it is aggravated by movement, the patient usually lies quite still.

Patients with acute appendicitis provide a good illustration of these two types of pain. In the early stages when there is obstruction and consequent spasm in the appendix the patient has colicky pain vaguely referred to the area round the umbilicus, and he frequently vomits at the onset; but in a few hours, when inflammation has developed in the appendix and spread to involve the overlying parietal peritoneum, the pain becomes sharper and shifts to the right iliac fossa directly over the site of the lesion.

Pain and tenderness occur in the liver only when its capsule is acutely stretched by sudden distension of the organ, as in congestive cardiac failure; and in the spleen when there is inflammation of its peritoneal covering, as by an infarct extending to the surface.

Constipation

Few conditions are wrongly diagnosed more often than constipation. Many men and nearly all women when asked about their bowels reply that they have always tended to be rather constipated. They mean that instead of having a daily bowel action, which the patent-medicine advertisements have taught them is essential for normal health, their bowels move only once every two or three days. They have therefore fallen into the habit of taking a purgative every day or once or twice a week, and they believe that continuing with this ritual is essential to their well-being. In fact, however, variations in the normal rhythm of the colon are quite wide, and to evacuate the bowel twice a week is not constipation; it is just as normal and healthy as to evacuate it twice a day.

On the other hand, it must be recognised that when a patient with a lifelong addiction to purgatives is admitted to hospital with some organic complaint, the kindest and most sensible plan is to continue prescribing his usual laxative. The time is not appropriate to attempt re-education of bowel function, which in any case would be most unlikely to succeed.

A normal regular movement of the bowels is not to be expected in febrile dehydrated patients who are taking little or no solid food, and a dose of cascara or senna or a simple enema every few days is all that is needed. Greater care must be taken to ensure a regular evacuation in weak, elderly patients, in whom impaction of a mass of faeces in the rectum tends to occur.

Diarrhoea

Acute diarrhoea is usually due to dietetic indiscretion, food poisoning, infections such as bacillary dysentery, or an exacerbation in one of the causes of chronic diarrhoea.

Chronic diarrhoea may arise from:

1 **the stomach,** as a result of achlorhydria or after gastrectomy or vagotomy,

2 **the small intestine,** in patients with regional ileitis (Crohn's disease) or a malabsorption syndrome such as sprue,

3 **the colon,** from carcinoma, diverticulitis, amoebic dysentery or ulcerative colitis.

Apart from alimentary disorders such as the above, chronic diarrhoea may be due to general causes, such as thyrotoxicosis or anxiety neurosis.

Vomiting

Vomiting is produced by compression of the stomach between the muscles of the abdominal wall and the diaphragm, with simultaneous relaxation of the cardiac sphincter. The causes are very numerous, but fall into a few main groups:

1 When due to **intra-abdominal disease** it is usually preceded by nausea. In pyloric obstruction the vomiting may be projectile, the gastric contents being ejected from the patient's mouth with great force, and frequently very large quantities of vomit are produced containing recognisable food taken many hours previously. In intestinal obstruction the reverse peristalsis throughout the gut may eventually cause faeculent vomiting.

2 **Cerebral vomiting** occurs in patients with raised intracranial pressure, and there is often no preceding nausea. Disturbances of the balance mechanism in the labyrinth of the inner ear are also common causes of vomiting, as in patients with acute vertigo or travel sickness.

3 **Psychological vomiting** is also common. Some people vomit from sudden fear or horror, as for example if they see an accident in the street; others do so for less obvious and more deep-seated psychological reasons. Frequently repeated persistent vomiting without loss of weight is nearly always of this type.

Diseases of the Oesophagus

The commonest symptom arising in the oesophagus is difficulty in swallowing (dysphagia). In young people dysphagia is most likely to be due to the condition known as achalasia of the cardia; after middle age carcinoma of the oesophagus is the more probable diagnosis. Substernal burning pain is the only other common symptom arising in the oesophagus, and it is often due to irritation of the mucous membrane by acid which has regurgitated from the stomach through a cardiac sphincter made incompetent by the presence of a hiatus hernia (see p. 82).

Achalasia of the Cardia (Cardiospasm)

The word 'achalasia' means 'failure to relax', and it was coined by Hurst because he believed that this was the explanation for the obstruction to the passage of food through the cardiac sphincter. The oesophagus becomes greatly distended and elongated. The patient complains that his food sticks at the level of the lower end of the sternum and he has a feeling of discomfort and fullness in the chest after meals. Food residue in the oesophagus may find its way into the air passages during sleep and give rise to symptoms of lung abscess or bronchiectasis.

The **diagnosis** is confirmed by barium swallow under X-ray screening, which shows a greatly dilated oesophagus which has to be filled to a height of several inches before any barium will pass through into the stomach.

Treatment Octyl nitrite 0.2 ml in a glass capsule which is broken into a handkerchief and inhaled relaxes the cardia but this effect lasts for only 2 minutes and treatment giving more permanent relief is always needed. Dilatation with an instrument such as the Starke dilator is often very effective. If this fails, or if the gullet is obviously dilated, cardiomyotomy (Heller's operation) should be performed. Results are excellent except in patients with gross dilatation and tortuosity of the gullet, who require more extensive surgical procedures.

Carcinoma of the Oesophagus

This is commoner in men than in women. The first complaint is that solid foods tend to stick at the level of the growth (which is usually halfway down the oesophagus or at its lower end). At first semisolid food can be swallowed normally, but as the obstruction becomes more complete even fluids may fail to go down. The other striking clinical feature is extremely rapid loss of weight. The diagnosis is confirmed by barium swallow and by oesophagoscopy, which enables a small piece of tumour to be removed for histological examination. The treatment is entirely surgical.

The Plummer-Vinson (Paterson Brown-Kelly) Syndrome

This is a cause of dysphagia in middle-aged women. These women have no acid in the stomach (achlorhydria), which impairs the absorption of iron from the food, and usually in addition their diet has been deficient in the expensive iron-containing foods, such as meat and green vegetables, and they have a history of excessive loss of iron through menstruation and pregnancy. In consequence severe iron deficiency develops, leading to hypochromic anaemia (see p. 33) and to atrophy of the mucous membrane of the tongue, which becomes smooth and sore, and of the pharynx and upper oesophagus, causing dysphagia. The condition can be cured quite readily by giving iron. It is very important that this should be done, for if the iron deficiency is allowed to persist, carcinoma of the upper end of the oesophagus may develop as a complication.

Hiatus Hernia

This is not of course primarily an oesophageal disorder, but it may conveniently be considered here, since the resulting symptoms are entirely due to oesophagitis. The hiatus in question is the hole in the diaphragm through which the oesophagus passes before joining the fundus of the stomach. When hiatus hernia occurs, part of the stomach is forced up through this hole in the diaphragm into the thorax; if the lower end of the oesophagus remains in its normal place and the herniated portion of stomach lies alongside it in the thorax the latter is called a para-oesophageal hernia, but if the oesophagus is pushed bodily upwards through the diaphragm by the herniating stomach the term 'sliding hernia' is used. In either type of hiatus hernia the important point is that the cardiac sphincter no longer works efficiently, so that when the stomach is compressed after a meal (as for example by the patient bending down), and also when he lies flat in bed, gastric contents regurgitate freely into the oesophagus. Now, the lining of the stomach is designed by nature to resist the action of acid, but the lining of the oesophagus is not, and in consequence it becomes inflamed when it is brought frequently into contact with hydrochloric acid from the stomach.

The main **symptom** of hiatus hernia, therefore, is burning pain felt high in the epigastrium and behind the sternum, often troubling the patient particularly when he stoops or takes active exercise soon after a meal and when he lies in bed at night.

Treatment The patient is advised to avoid those activities which encourage gastric contents to pass into the oesophagus; he should not stoop or take exercise for an hour or so after eating and he should raise the head of his bed on blocks about 18 cm high. He is given an antacid, in tablet form or powder form, to neutralise any acid which does reach the oesophagus; and Gaviscon sachets chewed and washed down with water after meals may prevent acid reflux by forming a 'raft' which floats on the gastric contents. In spite of these medical measures, however, some patients continue to have symptoms, and for them surgical repair of the hiatus hernia usually gives very satisfactory results.

Gastritis

Gastritis means inflammation of the stomach, and it is a term often used rather loosely to explain dyspeptic symptoms for which a more satisfactory pathological cause cannot be found.

Acute Gastritis is due to an irritant such as excessive alcohol or food poisoning, or occasionally to an acute specific infection such as influenza. The symptoms are loss of appetite, nausea, vomiting and abdominal discomfort; diarrhoea often occurs too, due to an associated enteritis (inflammation of the intestines). The symptoms subside spontaneously in a few days, and all that is needed in the way of treatment is to keep the patient warm and comfortable and avoid any further irritation of his stomach.

Chronic Gastritis in its most typical form is due to chronic alcoholism. The patient complains of loss of appetite and nausea, particularly in the early morning, and often vomits mucus which has collected in the oesophagus and stomach during the night. He does not feel well until he has had another drink or two (a 'hair of the dog that bit him'), and so the vicious circle goes on. The only treatment of any value is complete and permanent abstention from alcohol. Chronic inflammation of the stomach occurs less often in people who are not alcoholics, and its cause is not known. In many patients diagnosed as having chronic gastritis the symptoms are probably mainly of psychological origin.

Peptic Ulcer

A peptic ulcer is a hole in the mucous membrane of the stomach or the first part of the duodenum. These are the only parts of the alimentary tract in which the contents are acid in reaction, since the bile and pancreatic juices flowing into the second part of the duodenum are strongly alkaline. Normally the mucous membrane of the stomach and first part of the duodenum can resist the action of the hydrochloric acid; what renders it susceptible to erosion in patients with peptic ulcer remains a mystery. In other words, the cause of gastric and duodenal ulcer is still unknown.

A few general comments can be made, however. Some people seem to inherit a tendency to peptic ulcer, which is very common in some families and uncommon in others. The sex incidence of gastric ulcers is almost equal; duodenal ulcers are 3–4 times more common in men than in women. In Western countries gastric and duodenal ulcer now seem to be significantly more common in poor people. Patients with duodenal ulcer have twice as many acid-secreting cells in their gastric mucosa as normal people or patients with gastric ulcer. There is no firm evidence that psychological factors, physique or personality are important in the cause of ulcer, but anxiety, overwork and stress of various kinds often lead to exacerbation of symptoms.

Peptic ulcer has a natural tendency to heal and then recur, and the relapses often come at times when the patient is overworked or faced with great personal difficulties. There is also a seasonal incidence: most sufferers find that their symptoms are particularly likely to return in unpleasant cold weather in the late autumn or early spring. The disease is very common in early adult life and middle age, less common in old age, and very rare in childhood.

Symptoms The main symptom is pain in the epigastrium related to the taking of food. With duodenal ulcer it is a hunger pain and disappears for 2 or 3 hours after a meal; with gastric ulcer the pain usually comes on ½ to 1 hour after meals and is not so strikingly relieved by eating. The pain is also temporarily eased by taking alkali or by vomiting. A very important symptom in patients with duodenal ulcer is pain waking them up about 2 or 3 a.m.

Great stress should be laid on a history of remissions in the symptoms; a patient who has had pain or other dyspeptic symptoms for a year or more without any intervals of freedom is very unlikely to have a peptic ulcer.

Signs The pointing test is the most helpful sign: when asked to indicate where he has the pain, the patient points with his finger to the middle of the epigastrium. Tenderness in the epigastrium may also be found.

Investigations The diagnosis is confirmed by barium meal, which means examination by an experienced radiologist after the patient has swallowed sufficient barium to make his stomach and duodenum visible on the X-ray screen. The fibre-optic endoscope is a flexible instrument which is passed into the stomach and duodenum and enables an expert to see the ulcer and if necessary take a biopsy from its base.

It is usual also for the stools to be examined for occult (or hidden) blood. Some bleeding always occurs when the ulcer is active, and although the amount of blood passing through the intestines is insufficient to alter the normal colour of the faeces, its presence can be detected by chemical tests. False positive results may be obtained if the patient has recently eaten meat, which must therefore be excluded from the patient's diet for 3 days before the specimen of stool is sent to the laboratory. A disadvantage of this test is that a very small trace of blood, too little to be of clinical significance, may give a positive result. On the other hand, if tests for occult blood in the stools are repeatedly strongly positive, either the patient's peptic ulcer is active or he has some other bleeding lesion in the alimentary tract.

Complications

(1) Haemorrhage As pointed out above, a certain amount of bleeding always takes place from the raw surface of the ulcer, but sometimes when the ulcer is a deep one it erodes into an artery in the wall of the stomach or duodenum. Massive haemorrhage then occurs, and is a very serious complication. The patient may vomit a large quantity of blood (this is called a haematemesis), and it is obvious at once that serious bleeding is in progress, but if the blood goes the other way down through the intestines, the diagnosis must be made first on the signs of internal haemorrhage and later on the appearance of a large amount of altered blood in the stools making them black and tarry. The latter event is known as a melaena. Internal haemorrhage should be suspected in a patient who complains of sudden faintness and is found on examination to be pale and sweating, with a fast, thready pulse and a low blood pressure.

(2) Perforation This means that the ulcer has eaten its way through the whole thickness of the wall of the stomach or duodenum and in consequence the very irritant acid contents leak out into the peritoneal cavity. The patient immediately complains of severe generalised abdominal pain. He lies quite still because any movement aggravates his pain; he shows signs of shock (pallor, sweating, tachycardia and low blood pressure); and his abdominal muscles are found to be in a state of rigid spasm. The diagnosis is usually easily made from this striking clinical picture and an emergency operation to close the perforation should be done without delay.

(3) Pyloric Stenosis This is a complication of duodenal ulcer situated just beyond the pyloric sphincter. Through the years fibrous tissue is laid down in the base of the ulcer in an attempt at healing, and as fibrous tissue always undergoes contraction in the course of time, the first part of the duodenum may become seriously constricted. Consequently the food and gastric juices in the stomach find increasing difficulty in passing through into the duodenum. The stomach becomes distended and is evacuated from time to time by vomiting; if the vomit contains recognisable items of food, such as tomato skins, known to have been eaten more than a few hours before, it provides clear evidence of delay in gastric emptying and probably of pyloric stenosis. Patients with pyloric stenosis lose weight and become dehydrated, and from the loss of certain salts through vomiting they may develop a variety of muscular irritability known as tetany. This gives rise to painful spasm in the muscles of the arms and legs (carpopedal spasms). Compression of the upper arm by the sphygmomanometer cuff may cause the limb to go into spasm; this is known as Trousseau's sign of latent tetany. The abdomen is generally sunken and the skin loose, but the distended stomach may cause a bulge in the left upper quadrant, and the peristaltic efforts it is making to force its contents through the stenosed pylorus may be seen as a ripple passing across from left to right. The only satisfactory *treatment* for pyloric stenosis is gastrojejunostomy, an operation making an artificial opening between the stomach and jejunum by which food can by-pass the obstruction in the duodenum.

The Treatment of Peptic Ulcer

The object in medical treatment is to promote conditions in which the ulcer will heal, and the most important of these are rest and abstaining from smoking.

Generally speaking the patient will be allowed up morning and evening for washing and toilet purposes, but otherwise be confined to bed in the early stages. This is necessary not only for the beneficial effect of complete physical rest, but also because such confinement helps to shield him from mental stimulation and worry. This psychological aspect must always be considered carefully and with common sense. Some men worry more if they cannot keep in touch with their business by telephone or see a colleague occasionally. The aim is to achieve physical and mental relaxation, and the nurse must always be thinking of the best way of doing this, having regard to the particular temperament and personality of her patient. To help in calming a very active and restless mind, a tranquilliser may be prescribed, such as diazepam (Valium) 2 mg two or three times daily.

Diet The present tendency is not to insist on such rigid dietary regimes as used to be enforced. The general principle is that small bland meals are given at frequent intervals; long gaps between feeds in particular must be avoided, since it is when the stomach is empty that irritation of the ulcer and pain mostly occur.

In view of this the nurse must ensure that drinks are given at the correct time. This type of patient tends to keep one eye on the clock and is easily upset when feeds are late.

Nearly all patients with peptic ulcer lose their pain when they have been in bed for a few days, but for those whose pain is unusually severe and persistent the milk 'drip' method is a useful form of treatment. A tube is passed into the stomach, preferably through the nose, and connected to a milk container above the bed. The flow is adjusted to a slow drip by means of a clip so that the patient receives some 3 litres in the course of 24 hours. This procedure is often remarkably effective in relieving previously intractable pain.

Suggested Gastric Diets

Stage 1 (to be given while the patient has symptoms): Frequent milky feeds supplemented by strained gruel, junkets, jellies, baked custard, milk soup containing purée or vegetables, bread and butter, purée of potato (if permitted), a little sugar and half a teaspoon of salt daily given with soup feeds.

Stage 2 (To be given when patient has recently become free from symptoms): Add—weak, milky tea; lightly boiled, poached or scrambled eggs; white fish, chicken, sweetbreads or brains; purée of potato and purée of vegetables; purée of fruit and fruit juices, unless they produce pain; a little finely minced meat; sponge cake, a plain biscuit and any light sweet which is smooth in consistency.

However, there is no evidence that special diets do more than help to relieve the symptoms of peptic ulcer; in particular, it has not been shown that they promote healing or prevent relapse of the ulcer, so that when the patient has been free of symptoms for a week or two he may be allowed a normal diet, avoiding only those items he knows by experience may upset him.

The patient's teeth should be examined and any necessary treatment carried out as soon as possible. While he is having a more or less fluid diet chewing-gum or barley sugars will encourage the flow of saliva and so keep the mouth fresh and clean. When taking solid food the patient should be taught the importance of good mastication.

Cimetidine (Tagamet) is very effective in reducing the secretion of acid and is the drug of first choice for gastric and duodenal ulcer; it gives symptomatic relief and promotes healing. It is given in doses of 200 mg t.d.s. with 400 mg at bedtime for 6 weeks followed by 400 mg at night for up to a year. Ranitidine is a drug with similar effects and may be used as an alternative.

Antacids Traditionally antacids such as aluminium hydroxide and magnesium trisilicate have been given for symptomatic relief of pain. More recently it has been shown that when given in large doses at particular times antacids also promote healing of duodenal, but not gastric, ulcers. For this purpose a combination of aluminium and magnesium hydroxide (Maalox) may be given, 10–30 ml one hour and three hours after meals.

Antispasmodics Drugs of the belladonna group, which paralyse the vagus nerves, are given to reduce the increased motor activity of the stomach, which is probably one of the factors causing pain and preventing healing of the ulcer. They also reduce that part of the secretion of gastric juice which is stimulated by vagal impulses. Poldine (Nacton) is a suitable preparation; the initial dose, 2 mg three times daily, should be slowly increased until the patient notices slight dryness of the mouth.

Carbenoxolone has been proved effective in promoting the healing of gastric ulcers. It is given by mouth in doses of 100 mg t.d.s. and is avoided in patients with cardiac insufficiency, as it causes sodium and water retention.

Bowels The prescribed diet contains little or no roughage, and, as bowel movement may be sluggish, liquid paraffin or milk of magnesia may be necessary.

Duration of Treatment Even under favourable conditions healing of the ulcer will not occur in less than four to six weeks, though the patient is likely to be free of symptoms after the first few days. Ideally the period of strict treatment should continue for some two weeks after the ulcer can no longer be demonstrated by barium meal. Before the patient is discharged he is told the importance of following a certain regime and given written instructions for reference. He must have regular meals, he must not go more than 2½ hours without a small meal or milk drink, and a glass of milk and biscuits should be kept by the bedside. The patient himself will find which food suits him best and with care many patients are able to take an almost normal diet. Alcohol before meals should be avoided, but a very moderate amount of beer or light wine may be taken with a meal. Smoking is best avoided. Alkalies may be taken to relieve pain, but the recurrence of this symptom should be reported to the doctor.

Surgical treatment for peptic ulcer is much safer than it used to be and is consequently more frequently employed. It is even more frequently demanded by the patient himself, who naturally thinks that if only he can have his ulcer cut out that will be the end of it and he need have no more tedious weeks in hospital and irksome diets. Unfortunately, however, the matter is not as simple as this. The operations performed are either vagotomy with pyloroplasty (cutting the vagus nerve to reduce acid secretion with a plastic operation which improves gastric emptying) or partial gastrectomy (which removes part of the acid-secreting stomach). Many patients do very well after operation, but persistent diarrhoea is common after vagotomy and some who have had gastrectomy develop troublesome distension and faintness after meals, and anaemia from impaired iron absorption develops in about 30% of them. It would be wrong therefore to advise operation indiscriminately for patients with peptic ulcer. Surgery should, however, be considered for a patient whose ulcer has (1) failed to heal after a period of efficient medical treatment, (2) caused pyloric obstruction, (3) caused severe bleeding, particularly if this has occurred more than once and if the patient is above middle age. It may be advisable to operate on a patient with a gastric ulcer even before he has been treated medically if there is doubt that the ulcer may be malignant; duodenal ulcers are never malignant. It has already been pointed out that perforation is an immediate indication for operation.

The Treatment of Massive Bleeding A patient who has had a large haematemesis or melaena is always an anxious and difficult problem in treatment, demanding great care and skill on the part of both medical and nursing staff. In the hope that the bleeding will stop spontaneously he must be kept as quiet as possible; an injection of morphine 15–20 mg is therefore given on admission and repeated in a few hours if he becomes restless. Blood is taken for haemoglobin estimation and grouping and an hourly pulse and blood pressure chart is started. Transfusion may not be necessary if the patient is young and the haemorrhage relatively slight, but an elderly patient who had bled severely must be given a litre of blood without delay. It used to be thought that transfusion might be dangerous by re-starting the bleeding, but there is no doubt that the risk of withholding blood from an exsanguinated patient is much greater. Continuing internal haemorrhage is shown by a rising pulse-rate and falling blood pressure, and these are therefore also indications for transfusion. At one time these patients were given only ice to suck in the early stages, in the mistaken idea that this would rest the stomach. It is well known, however, that an empty stomach is in fact much more active than a full one, and it is wiser to give the patient a diet corresponding to the first stage of the usual peptic ulcer regime as soon as he can take it. Operation may be needed if the bleeding continues or recurs, but carries a high mortality in these severely ill patients; so that in some cases to decide correctly whether surgery or conservative treatment is the more dangerous is extremely difficult. Fortunately, bleeding to this extent is relatively uncommon; in most patients the haemorrhage does stop spontaneously and their further treatment is that of uncomplicated peptic ulcer, with the addition of the iron therapy which is needed to make up the blood which has been lost.

Carcinoma of the Stomach

Carcinoma of the stomach is one of the commonest forms of cancer in men. Early diagnosis is of the utmost importance if the patient is to have any chance of radical cure, and to this end the possibility of malignant disease of the stomach should always be considered when a man above about the age of 45 develops for the first time dyspeptic symptoms which do not respond to treatment within two or three weeks. The symptoms are very variable, but the commonest are loss of appetite and epigastric pain not usually closely related to the taking of food. Within a few months loss of weight and evidence of anaemia become obvious. Frequently a good deal of bleeding occurs from the surface of the carcinoma and the vomiting of altered blood which looks like coffee-grounds is a characteristic feature. Sometimes the growth causes obstruction at the pylorus, producing symptoms and signs similar to those of pyloric stenosis (see p. 86); less often it is situated at the cardia, obstructing the opening of the oesophagus into the stomach, and the patient complains that his food seems to stick at the level of the lower end of the sternum. In some unfortunate patients the earliest symptoms are those due to secondary deposits in the liver or elsewhere.

In advanced cases a hard, fixed mass can be felt in the epigastrium. At an earlier stage the diagnosis is made usually on the result of the barium meal examination followed by endoscopy: this involves passing into the stomach a fibre-optic instrument through which the lesion can be seen and a portion removed for histological proof of the diagnosis.

Treatment Unhappily the prognosis of carcinoma of the stomach is extremely bad. In only a small proportion of the patients is it found possible to perform a radical operation for the removal of the growth, and of them only a few survive for 5 years after the operation. For the majority of patients, therefore, the problem is to keep them as comfortable as possible in the few months that remain. If pyloric obstruction occurs, a palliative short-circuit operation should certainly be done to relieve the copious vomiting, rapid wasting and dehydration, and if anaemia becomes severe a transfusion will bring a temporary improvement in general strength. Chlorpromazine (Largactil), given either intramuscularly or by mouth in doses of 25–50 mg three times daily, often helps to relieve nausea and vomiting and to reduce mental tension and distress, and when pain becomes troublesome pethidine or opium derivatives must be given in adequate doses. Pethidine 50–100 mg intramuscularly may be tried first, and if morphine 15–20 mg causes sickness, heroin 8–10 mg is a useful alternative; the dosage must of course be increased as tolerance develops. Most important of all is a calm, efficient and cheerful nurse who has gained the full confidence of her patient.

Jaundice

Physiology of Bile Red corpuscles in the blood wear out in about 120 days, after which time they are removed from the circulation and broken up by special cells situated in the bone-marrow, the liver and the spleen. In the breaking-up process the haemoglobin is split into two fractions, an iron-containing part which is returned to the bone-marrow to be built into new red corpuscles, and a non-iron-containing part from which a pigment called bilirubin is liberated into the blood. Normal blood therefore always contains a certain amount of this bile pigment, in a form in which it is insoluble in water and unable to escape through the glomerular filters of the kidney into the urine. When it reaches the liver, however, the liver cells remove it from the plasma proteins and secrete it into the biliary passages, through which it flows, together with the bile salts also derived from the liver, into the duodenum. In the duodenum the bilirubin is converted into urobilinogen, which is the pigment responsible for most of the normal colour of the faeces. A little of this urobilinogen is absorbed from the small intestine into the portal bloodstream; and though nearly all of this fraction is removed again by the liver cells and returned to the biliary passages, traces of it sometimes escape through the liver into the general circulation and are excreted in the urine.

Definition of Jaundice Jaundice is an increase in the amount of bilirubin in the blood which, when it rises above a certain level, causes a yellow discoloration to appear in the skin and the sclerotics of the eyes.

Causes of Jaundice It will be obvious from the above discussion that jaundice may result either because too much bilirubin is liberated into the blood from the breakdown of more red corpuscles than normal (haemolytic jaundice), or because too little bilirubin is removed from the blood in its passage through the liver. The latter disorder can come about in two ways: either because an obstruction in the common bile duct dams the flow of bile, and bilirubin removed by the liver cells from the incoming blood, having no outlet, simply diffuses back into the blood (obstructive jaundice); or because the liver cells are sick and unable to perform their normal function of removing the bilirubin from the blood (hepatic jaundice).

Haemolytic Jaundice

This is the least common of the three main types of jaundice, and the yellow discoloration of the skin and other tissues is never more than slight. The urine contains no bilirubin, since, as explained above, the bilirubin is attached to the plasma proteins, which hold it in the blood and prevent its passing through the glomerular filters of the kidney. Since more bile pigment than normal is being produced, an excess of urobilinogen is formed from it in the intestine; for this reason the stools retain their normal colour (indeed, chemical analysis would show that they contain an excess of urobilinogen), and an excess of urobilinogen is found also in the urine.

The familial disease acholuric jaundice is the best example of a haemolytic jaundice. These patients have abnormally fragile red blood corpuscles, which are destroyed (or haemolysed) long before the normal span of 120 days. Removal of the enlarged spleen usually gives very satisfactory results.

Obstructive Jaundice

Patients with complete obstruction of the common bile duct become more and more deeply jaundiced and may eventually acquire a dark olive-green colour. They also frequently complain of irritation of the skin. Since no bile is reaching the duodenum, no urobilinogen is formed; for this reason the stools lose their pigment and become putty coloured, and no urobilinogen is present in the urine. On the other hand, the bilirubin in the blood of these patients passes freely into the urine; this may be partly because there is so much more of it than in patients with haemolytic jaundice, but mainly because after passing through the liver cells it becomes soluble in water. Whatever the theoretical explanation, the practical point is that the urine is dark in colour, shows a greenish froth when shaken, and chemical tests (such as Fouchet's) show that bilirubin is present. The two commonest causes of obstructive jaundice are gall-stones in the common bile duct and carcinoma of the head of the pancreas compressing its lower end.

Hepatic Jaundice

This is seen in patients whose liver has been seriously damaged, usually only temporarily, by infections such as virus hepatitis or poisons such as chloroform. Obstruction to the bile ducts which lie within the liver usually occurs at some stage of the illness and is shown by the appearance of putty-coloured stools and bilirubin in the urine.

Infectious Hepatitis

Infection with Virus A has an incubation period of about a month. The virus is present in the patient's stools, and the infection is usually acquired as the result of contamination of food or water. In this country only sporadic cases are seen, but where large groups of people are living under relatively primitive conditions in a warm climate widespread epidemics may occur. Thus, during the war there were large outbreaks among troops in India and the Middle East. Under these conditions flies are important agents in the spread of the infection. Virus infection may also be transmitted by homosexual men.

On recovery the patient is nearly always immune from further attacks. Furthermore, there is some evidence to suggest that the virus of infective hepatitis causes only a mild gastro-enteritis in young children and that those who acquire the more severe illness in adult life are those who have escaped childhood infection and consequent immunisation. This is known to apply to some other virus infections, such as poliomyelitis, which are more serious in adults than in children.

Serum Hepatitis (or B virus infection) has a longer incubation period (about 3 months) and infection is acquired through transfusions or injections containing serum. B virus antigen may be found in the blood of these patients and as some healthy people harbour the virus in their blood for long periods, anyone found to be B virus positive should be excluded from service as a blood donor. This infection is a particular hazard in dialysis units treating patients with chronic renal failure.

Non-A Non-B Viral Hepatitis This virus has not been isolated but its occurrence is assumed from epidemiological evidence. It causes an illness similar to B virus hepatitis and is responsible for many cases of chronic active hepatitis.

Clinical Features The illness starts with fever, general malaise, aching in the back and limbs, nausea and loss of appetite. After a few days the patient becomes jaundiced, the liver is found to be enlarged and slightly tender and occasionally the spleen is palpable. In the first few days the urine contains an excess of urobilinogen; then when intra-hepatic biliary obstruction occurs the urobilinogen disappears and bilirubin is found in the urine; and finally, after bilirubin has disappeared there may be a temporary return of urobilinogen before the urine reverts to normal. The great majority of patients are jaundiced for only a week or two, and then make a complete recovery. Very occasionally, however, the infection damages the liver so severely that death occurs within a few days from hepatic failure; or, equally rarely, recovery is not complete and slowly progressive damage to the liver eventually leads to cirrhosis.

Treatment There is no specific treatment for infective hepatitis but recently a vaccine has been produced which may be effective in preventing B virus infection. The most important measure undoubtedly is complete rest; and as a general rule the patient should be kept in bed until the temperature has settled, his appetite has returned, bilirubin has disappeared from his urine and his liver is no longer tender.

Because the virus is present in the stools, particular care should be taken in the disposal of excreta and the washing of hands after attending the patient.

Occasionally irritation of the skin may be troublesome, due to the bile salts, but it can usually be relieved by keeping the patient cool and applying soothing lotions.

Because of the loss of appetite, the patient is at first able to take only sweetened fruit drinks, tea with lemon or very little milk, and Bovril; the smell of food is often sufficient to cause nausea.

When the appetite begins to return there is usually a distaste for fats. Nothing is to be gained by forcing unwelcome food, and a low fat diet should be continued as long as the patient wishes. On the other hand, a high protein intake should be ensured as soon as possible for repair of damaged liver cells. It is probably wise to give a supplement of B group vitamins.

The very nature of the disease causes irritability and often periods of depression, so that understanding, reassurance and help on the part of the nurse are very important. The patient may not wish to see visitors and may burst into tears for no apparent reason. Insomnia will aggravate this symptom, and sleep must be encouraged by ascertaining that the patient is comfortable. Drugs normally detoxicated by the liver, for example morphine and barbiturates, are best avoided, since their effects may be dangerously profound and prolonged. For the same reason alcohol should not be taken during the attack and for several weeks afterwards.

The patient may complain of not having any energy and feeling depressed for some time, and an adequate period of convalescence is essential.

Cirrhosis of the Liver

This is a diffuse and progressive fibrosis of the liver which may arise in a number of different ways. Quite often the cause is not known.

Biliary cirrhosis occurs in patients with long-standing or recurrent obstruction of the common bile duct from gall-stones; stasis in the biliary passages leads to chronic or recurrent infection and results in the laying down of fibrous tissue throughout the liver.

Multilobular or Portal Cirrhosis (Laennec's cirrhosis), is commoner but frequently more obscure. There is an undoubted relationship between chronic alcoholism and cirrhosis, but on the other hand the disease sometimes affects teetotallers. In the alcoholic variety there is usually a history of epigastric discomfort, loss of appetite—particularly for breakfast—and morning sickness with vomiting of mucus, symptoms attributable to alcoholic gastritis; but patients with idiopathic cirrhosis have frequently had no symptoms up to the time of diagnosis. In this variety the cause of the disease is unknown; one theory suggests that these patients have a low-grade but persistent virus infection of the liver.

Clinical Features Whatever the cause of the disease, the final stage of diffuse hepatic fibrosis produces a fairly typical clinical picture. The symptoms and signs are due to two main causes:

1 **Portal Hypertension** Shortening of the fibrous tissue laid down throughout the liver leads to compression of blood vessels and impedes the blood flowing in through the portal vein. The pressure in the portal vein and its tributaries consequently rises, and as the normal route through the liver becomes more and more obstructed, the blood in the portal system has to find alternative pathways to the inferior vena cava and heart. The most important alternative pathway is via the veins at the lower end of the oesophagus, which become enormously distended; rupture of one of these veins, and consequent severe haematemesis, is therefore one of the most serious complications of cirrhosis. Other veins which may become abnor-

mally distended are those on the abdominal wall and in the rectum. The splenic vein is a tributary of the portal vein, and the spleen usually enlarges and becomes palpable in patients with portal hypertension.

2 **Impairment of the Various Functions of the Liver** One of the most interesting effects of impaired liver function is the development on the face, neck, arms and upper half of the trunk of lesions known as 'spider naevi'. These consist of a central red spot a millimetre or so in diameter with fine red lines radiating from it; pressure on the central spot causes the whole lesion to blanch. Erythema (redness) of the palms of the hands often occurs in the same patients. Both spider naevi and red palms are sometimes seen also in normal pregnancy.

Another important function of the liver is the manufacture and regulation of the various plasma proteins. In cirrhosis the concentration of plasma proteins is reduced, especially the albumin fraction, and there is therefore a fall in the osmotic pressure of the blood. Partly for this reason, and partly because of the portal hypertension described above, accumulation of fluid in the peritoneal cavity (ascites) is another important complication of cirrhosis. Whiteness of the nails (leuconychia) is sometimes seen in patients whose serum albumin level is very low.

In the final stages of cirrhosis, when impairment of liver function is very severe, jaundice may occur because of the failure of the liver-cells to remove bilirubin from the blood, and the patient may eventually pass into hepatic coma from the effect on the brain of toxic substances absorbed from the intestine which would normally have been destroyed by the liver.

Treatment Cirrhosis is at present an incurable disease, thus treatment can only be directed to the relief or prevention of its various ill-effects.

On the whole the outlook is rather better in patients with alcoholic cirrhosis, since in them the cause of the disease is known. If they abstain from alcohol completely and permanently and take an adequate amount of protein in their diet further liver damage is avoided, and if the disease is not yet in an advanced stage there may even be some recovery of function.

Patients with other forms of cirrhosis should also avoid alcohol. In the early stages a high protein diet should be given but when the disease is advanced and liver failure is imminent a high protein intake may induce hepatic coma, and the diet has to be adjusted accordingly.

Ascites can usually be relieved by a low-sodium diet and the powerful diuretic frusemide (Lasix) which is given by mouth in doses of 40–120 mg daily. The thiazide diuretics may precipitate hepatic coma, but spironolactone 400 mg by mouth four times daily may be given. This antagonises the action of aldosterone, the salt-retaining hormone of the adrenal cortex whose excessive production is partly responsible for the development of the ascites. If the ascites cannot be controlled by these measures the fluid has to be removed by tapping (paracentesis abdominis), but this should be avoided if possible.

Patients with severe portal hypertension, revealed by a haematemesis, and without evidence of serious impairment of liver function, may be considered for the operation of 'portocaval shunt'. This involves making a communication between the portal vein and the inferior vena cava to relieve the gross distension of the oesophageal veins and prevent further bleeding from them.

Patients in hepatic coma must be given enough calories as intravenous glucose to minimise the breakdown of tissue protein, if necessary through a catheter passed into the vena cava. Ammonium absorption from the gut is reduced by giving neomycin 1 g four times daily to kill the intestinal bacteria which form ammonia from protein, and an injection of pitressin may be given to cause evacuation of melaena stools (which, of course, contain much protein).

Sprue and Gluten Enteropathy

Steatorrhoea means fatty diarrhoea or the passage of excessive amounts of fat in the stools. It is the most prominent feature of both sprue and gluten enteropathy, which are clinically identical conditions; sprue occurs in people living in or recently returned from the tropics, particularly India, whereas gluten enteropathy (coeliac disease) arises in temperate climates such as that of the British Isles. Sprue is probably due to a change in the bacterial flora in the gut resulting from repeated intestinal infections; gluten enteropathy is the adult counterpart of coeliac disease and is due to intestinal intolerance to gluten, which is the protein fraction of wheat.

Symptoms and Signs Histological examination reveals absence or abnormality of the villi of the intestinal mucous membrane, which fails to absorb enough of certain essential food factors. The unabsorbed food, a large part of which is the fat, passes through into the faeces, which are consequently pale, greasy, frothy and very bulky; and since the whole gut is abnormally filled with this unabsorbed residue, the abdomen shows a generalised distension.

The other symptoms and signs are due to the body's lack of the various food factors which are not being absorbed. Shortage of calories leads to loss of weight; lack of iron, vitamin B12 and folic acid causes anaemia; lack of other factors in the vitamin B complex, particularly nicotinic acid, riboflavin and aneurin, causes a sore, red tongue, cracking at the junctions of the upper and lower lips (angular stomatitis) and occasionally peripheral neuritis; in long-standing cases lack of calcium and vitamin D may lead to softening of the bones (osteomalacia); and occasionally lack of vitamin K causes a tendency to bleeding. **Systemic complications** include arthritis, skin lesions and inflammation of the eye (particularly iritis).

Treatment Patients with gluten enteropathy usually respond to a gluten-free diet within a few weeks and they must be told they will probably have to avoid gluten for life. To obtain such a diet all foods normally made with wheat-flour must be made instead with corn-flour or soya-bean flour. Otherwise the diet must be low in fat and in starchy foods. In addition, the various accessory food factors whose absorption is defective must be given in liberal quantities; folic acid, 5–20 mg daily by mouth, seems to be particularly important and often helps to relieve the diarrhoea as well as the anaemia. Iron is given by mouth as ferrous sulphate tablets, 0.2–0.4 g three times daily, or intramuscularly if the haemoglobin is not rising satisfactorily after a week or two of oral treatment. Vitamin B12 is given by intramuscular injection, in doses of about 50 mg weekly. Vitamin B complex, vitamin D and vitamin K are given either by mouth or by injection when clinical signs of their deficiency are present.

Ulcerative Colitis

This is a serious and chronic disease of the colon and although temporary remission of symptoms is common, relapse nearly always follows after a variable interval of months or years and complete recovery is extremely rare. The cause of ulcerative colitis is unknown. Its acute stage is very similar to bacillary dysentery, which suggests that an infection might be responsible, but no specific organism has ever been isolated. Some authorities have been very struck by the personality of these patients, who are said to be extremely fussy, tidy, meticulous people, emotionally immature and showing an abnormal dependence on one or other parent, and it has been suggested that the changes in the bowel are secondary to some psychological disturbance. Other physicians take the view that these psychological factors simply aggravate the disease, or indeed that they are the result of it.

Clinical Features The disease usually starts in early adult life and is rather commoner in women than in men. The principal symptom is diarrhoea, which continues in some degree throughout the whole course of the illness. During acute relapses the stools are greatly increased in number and contain blood and mucus, abdominal pain is often severe, the temperature is raised and the patient becomes very weak and anaemic; in remissions the general health becomes more or less restored, but there is nearly always some persistent looseness of the stools. The severity of the disease varies greatly in different patients. There is an acute fulminating variety which makes the patient gravely ill, even moribund, within a few weeks; at the other end of the scale is a mild type which causes only relatively trivial inconvenience; and between these extremes the majority of patients require admission to hospital from time to time over many years and are always more or less severely disabled by their disease.

Complications Stricture of the bowel, perforation, severe haemorrhage and the development of carcinoma in the diseased colon are complications particularly to be feared in the younger patients with severe ulcerative colitis.

Treatment There is no specific therapy for ulcerative colitis, and owing to the chronic and distressing nature of the disease, the great pain and weakness it causes and the sometimes difficult and childish personality of the patient, its treatment calls for the highest degree of skill and patience from the nursing staff. During the acute stages undoubtedly the most important measure is a period of complete rest in bed. Since the illness is a long one and the final result may depend on how well the patient's general strength has been maintained, it is vitally important that she should have a diet which is high in total calories and in protein. The appetite is poor, however, so that great attention must be paid to ensure that the food is well prepared and attractively served, that it contains sufficient variety to tempt the palate and that the patient's particular likes and dislikes are observed. A milk-free diet is sometimes helpful. Fluids should be given cool or warm, as very cold or very hot drinks stimulate the bowel. Vitamin supplements should also be given. For the relief of anaemia fresh blood transfusion is the most effective treatment and in addition often seems to be of benefit to the patient's general condition. Iron, either by mouth or intravenously, and B12 injections are also often given. To control the diarrhoea tab. codeine phosphate 30–60 mg three or four times daily or diphenoxylate (Lomotil) tab. 2 three or four times daily are the most useful measures. It is now usual to give sulfasalazine 1 g four times daily, reducing later to twice daily, since this has been shown to reduce the incidence of relapse. Many patients improve greatly after a course of prednisolone (Predsol) suppositories b.d. or retention enemas at night. Only if severe symptoms persist in spite of the above treatment should steroid therapy be used; then prednisolone is given by mouth starting with 60 mg daily and gradually reducing the dose. A gratifying remission is often induced in this way, but relapse all too often follows and maintenance therapy with prednisolone in low dosage (preferably not more than 10 mg daily) is often necessary.

Finally, some patients require surgical treatment. Operation is clearly indicated when there is evidence of perforation, stricture or malignant disease of the bowel. In addition the general condition of patients with severe ulcerative colitis usually improves very strikingly after the operation of ileostomy, as a result of which the contents of the lower ileum are discharged through an opening in the abdominal wall, and so do not pass through the diseased colon at all. At the same time the diseased colon is removed. The disadvantages are that operation on such a gravely ill patient carries a certain risk and that the improvement in health is bought at the price of a permanent ileostomy, since only rarely can the ileum be joined later to the stump of the rectum. For many patients, however, this price is worth paying.

Nursing care Although in certain respects it may be thought advisable to nurse the patient in a single room, to give as much privacy as possible, it is even more important for her to have the company of other patients at times, and the activities in a general ward will give her added interests; sufficient privacy can be given by the use of cubicle curtains. The bed should be conveniently near the sluice, to facilitate the frequent use of bedpans.

The degree of emaciation may be severe, and a well-sprung bed with sorbo mattress is essential. The patient should be bathed in bed daily. Some days she will be able to do a certain amount for herself, and this should be encouraged. Other days the exhaustion will be such that the nurse must do everything for her. Skin over bony prominences will require great care, and frequent changing of position is necessary.

Ordinary oral hygiene should be sufficient to keep the mouth clean, except of course in a severely ill patient, when extra care will have to be taken.

The need for frequent bedpans, the fear of soiling the bed and awareness of the offensiveness of the stools will worry the patient. The right attitude on the part of the nurse in this respect is of paramount importance. A bedpan left in a special locker by the bedside may reassure the patient and relieve the anxiety and an airwick will remove unpleasant smells. Special soft tissue or cotton wool will be used in place of the usual toilet paper. The skin round the anus must be washed frequently or cleansed with olive oil and a protective cream such as zinc and castor oil generously applied. An accurate report must be made of the number and character of the stools and any associated pain. For laboratory examination the stools must be fresh.

The temperature, pulse and respirations will be taken and recorded 4-hourly in the acute phases and otherwise twice daily. The patient should be weighed twice weekly.

If ileostomy has been done, particular care must be taken to prevent erosion of the surrounding skin by digestive juices which are present in the fluid faeces. Unless an ileostomy bag has been put on in the operating theatre it is necessary to change the dressing each time the ileostomy works, and a suitable barrier cream should be liberally applied after thorough cleansing of the area.

As already mentioned, emotional instability is often present, and the nurse must be prepared to expect many changes of moods and emotional outbursts, which she must meet with calmness, kindly firmness and tact. Every effort must be made to stimulate the patient's interests in things other than herself. Occupational therapy and a good library service can be a great help. The Medical Social Worker may be able to help in relieving her of financial and other worries.

Carcinoma of the Colon

Carcinoma hardly ever occurs in the small intestine, but is a common disease of the colon in both sexes above middle age. The commonest parts of the bowel to be affected are the pelvic colon and rectum; cancer at this site causes partial obstruction, with alternating constipation and diarrhoea and colicky abdominal pains, and recurrent rectal bleeding. Less often carcinoma arises in the ascending colon, where it causes more general symptoms, such as loss of weight, anorexia and anaemia. On examination a hard mass may be felt through the abdominal wall, but since most of these cancers lie deep in the pelvis, they can usually be detected only by rectal examination or, if necessary, by sigmoidoscopy. The latter investigation is particularly important and must never be omitted when a patient above early middle age complains of alteration in bowel habit or rectal bleeding.

Treatment Surgical removal of the carcinoma is the only effective treatment, and fortunately is much more often successful than in patients with carcinoma of the stomach.

Diverticular Disease

Diverticula of the colon are extremely common, particularly in fat elderly people; their presence is denoted by the term diverticulosis, a condition which causes no symptoms whatever. Symptoms arise only when the diverticula become inflamed; this is the disease known as diverticulitis.

Each diverticulum is a little hernia of the mucous membrane through the muscular wall of the bowel, and inflammation probably occurs in it as a result of constipation and the impaction of hard faecal material in its mouth.

Symptoms and Signs Colicky abdominal pain, particularly on the left side of the abdomen, fever and constipation are the main symptoms. On examination, a tender mass can usually be felt in relation to the affected part of the colon. A barium enema showing diverticula arising from the colon simply indicates diverticulosis; when diverticulitis is present there is narrowing and rigidity of the inflamed segment of bowel.

Complications Suppuration round an inflamed diverticulum may lead to abscess formation, and this may rupture into another organ, particularly the bladder (causing a vesicocolic fistula), or into the peritoneum, causing peritonitis.

Treatment Acute diverticulitis usually responds to a course of penicillin or other antibiotic. Diverticular disease is rare in countries where the staple diet is a high-residue one; a high-fibre diet (p. 226) should therefore be given, perhaps with the addition of bran 1–3 tablespoonsful daily. Operation is indicated only when the disease is complicated by intestinal obstruction, peritonitis or fistula.

6

The Urinary System

The Kidneys

Anatomy and Physiology

The kidneys are made up of several million microscopic units known as nephrons, each of which consists of a filter (the glomerulus) and a tubule. The blood supply to the kidneys passes first through the filters, and a fluid known as the glomerular filtrate diffuses from it into the tubules. The glomerular filtrate is a fluid whose composition is very similar to blood plasma, except that it contains no protein or fat; the tubules do not simply conduct it to the pelvis of the kidney but perform the very complex function of transforming it into urine. They do this by re-absorbing into the blood large amounts of water and other substances which the body needs to retain, and by secreting into it other substances which the body needs to excrete.

Renal Failure

Acute Renal Failure

Acute renal failure is a serious condition with a mortality of about 30 per cent. The exact cause is not known but factors certainly implicated are:

1 Sustained hypotension from haemorrhage, shock, etc.

2 Free circulating haemoglobin—usually from mismatched transfusion.

3 Extensive tissue damage.

4 Septicaemia—particularly with *E. coli* and staphylococci.

5 Renal disease, including acute glomerulonephritis, renal tract infection or obstruction.

Clinical Features The urinary output falls below 700 ml/24 hours and urea and potassium released from cell breakdown accumulate in the blood. The patient becomes sleepy and stuporose and nausea and vomiting are frequent. The chief danger is cardiac arrest from the elevated blood potassium level (hyperkalaemia). The low urine output of renal failure must be distinguished from **retention of urine,** if necessary by catheterisation, and from **dehydration** in which state the specific gravity of the urine is much higher (above 1015).

The low urinary output (oliguria) persists for up to 3 weeks and in patients who recover is followed by a diuretic phase in which huge volumes of dilute urine are passed. The danger now is excess loss of water, sodium and potassium. Slowly the urine volume and composition return to normal as tubular function recovers.

Treatment Throughout both phases the patient is highly susceptible to intercurrent infection, so barrier precautions are observed and he is given 500 000 units benzylpenicillin daily.

In the **oliguric phase** fluid and electrolyte loss must be replaced but over-hydration avoided. Sufficient calories must be given to minimise tissue breakdown and the release of urea and potassium into the blood. To achieve this at least 1500 Kcal should be given daily, so a high strength glucose solution containing 425 Kcal per 175 ml bottle (Hycal) is given by mouth in quantities equal to the fluid loss in the tears, breath and sweat; this is about 500 ml in the adult and may be increased to 1000 ml if the patient is feverish and sweating. If any urine is being passed the amount of glucose solution may be further increased by the volume of the urine output in the previous 24 hours. If vomiting is severe it may be necessary to give fluid as a 30% fructose solution intravenously through a polythene catheter every 24 hours. Tissue breakdown is further minimised by giving an anabolic steroid (norethandrolone 25 mg IM weekly). Rising plasma potassium levels may be temporarily controlled by adding 25 units of insulin to each bottle of 30% fructose, but if the level exceeds 7.5 mmol/litre (or the blood urea level exceeds 35 mmol/litre or the patient becomes increasingly drowsy) treatment by **dialysis** is necessary.

In the **diuretic phase,** which may develop very quickly, the aim is to replace the large amounts of water, sodium and potassium which are lost in the urine.

Nephritis

Nephritis may be defined as bilateral, non-suppurative diffuse disease of the kidneys and it presents as a number of syndromes each of which has several causes. These syndromes are **Acute Nephritis, Nephrotic Syndrome** and **Chronic Renal Failure.**

Acute Nephritis

Much the most common cause of this syndrome is acute glomerulonephritis which is probably an allergic reaction to a previous streptococcal infection. As a result of widespread damage to the glomeruli blood and protein leak into the urine.

Clinical Features The patient is usually a child or young adult who about one to three weeks after a streptococcal throat infection becomes suddenly ill with malaise, shivering and fever and sometimes pain in the loins or abdomen. The eyes become puffy and oedematous and the urine is scanty and bloodstained. About 90 per cent of these patients make a complete recovery, but in a few the symptoms and signs persist with increasing evidence of renal failure until they die usually within a year from uraemia and hypertension. Another small proportion make an apparently good recovery but continue to pass protein in the urine and may eventually develop either the nephrotic syndrome or chronic renal failure.

Treatment and Nursing Care Complete rest in bed is essential and must be continued until blood and protein have disappeared from the urine and when the patient is a child the nurse must exert great ingenuity to achieve this object. Excretion via the skin is encouraged by daily blanket baths and the patient's position must be changed four hourly and his pressure areas given frequent treatment. While fluids are restricted the mouth requires special care and frequent mouth-washes should be given. It is very important for the following observations to be recorded:

1 Daily urine volume.
2 Temperature and pulse chart.
3 Daily urine examination and measurement of its protein content.
4 Daily blood pressure.

In addition it is usual for the ESR to be estimated weekly.

The Diet should provide at least 1000 Kcal to prevent tissue breakdown and must be low in protein (less than 20–30 g/day) and salt. Such a diet consists of bread and butter (salt-free), jam, honey, cereals and fruit. Potatoes baked in their jackets or mashed with salt-free butter are a good source of calories. The most useful fluids are barley water, fruit drinks containing glucose, or weak tea with very little milk. At first fluids are restricted to 750 ml in 24 hours; as the urinary volume rises the fluid intake is increased. It is usual to give 500 ml plus a volume equal to that of the urine passed in the previous 24 hours. A diuresis usually occurs within a few days and then vegetables, milk, eggs, cheese and meat may be added to the diet.

Convalescence As the clinical state improves the patient should make a gradual return to full activity. Proteinuria may persist for up to a year and there is nothing to be gained by prolonging convalescence until it has entirely disappeared. On returning to normal life, chills and throat infections should be avoided as much as possible and streptococcal throat infections must be treated vigorously with antibiotics as they occur. Many physicians prescribe phenoxymethyl penicillin 250 mg daily by mouth for several years to prevent streptococcal throat infections and reduce the risk of further attacks of nephritis.

The Nephrotic Syndrome

The nephrotic syndrome is characterised by heavy proteinuria, low plasma proteins and oedema and its most common cause is the subacute variety of glomerulonephritis; other causes include diabetes mellitus, systemic lupus erythematosus and amyloid disease.

Clinical Features At first the patient has symptomless proteinuria, but when the plasma albumin drops below about 2 g/100 ml oedema gradually appears and slowly extends until finally it may affect the whole body. The face becomes pale and puffy, the legs show particularly severe distension and fluid may accumulate also in the peritoneal cavity, the pleural cavities and the pericardium. The urine usually contains more than 5 g protein in 24 hours. The course of the disease is variable, the oedema fluctuating in severity for weeks, months or even years, but ultimately the blood pressure and blood urea levels rise in most patients and they pass into chronic renal failure.

Treatment Patients with massive oedema have to be kept in bed but since rest probably does not influence the course of the disease, activity should be allowed as soon as oedema lessens sufficiently to make it possible. Since the oedema is due mainly to the loss of protein in the urine and the retention of sodium a diet high in protein and low in salt should be given. For reasons not fully understood steroid therapy sometimes leads to progressive decrease in proteinuria and oedema, particularly in children; it is usual therefore to give a trial of prednisolone, starting with 60 mg by mouth daily and reducing the dose by 10 mg every 5 days until a daily dose of 10 mg is reached. If the urine is now free of protein this dose is continued for three months and then tailed off. If protein persists the dose is adjusted and may be continued for longer periods.

Chronic Renal Failure

This may be the end result of many different diseases of the kidney, of which the most important is chronic glomerulonephritis. Other causes include chronic pyelonephritis, malignant hypertension, multiple renal stones, prostatic obstruction and diabetic nephropathy. Progressive damage to the nephrons eventually leads to the kidneys being unable to eliminate the waste products of metabolism, which consequently accumulate in the blood and lead to the clinical state known as **uraemia.**

Clinical Features. (*a*) **Early.** Insidious loss of energy is usually the first symptom and as the kidneys lose their ability to concentrate the urine the secretion of a larger volume of dilute urine disturbs the patient at night (nocturia). Examination reveals high blood pressure, and protein and granular casts in the urine and the blood urea level is raised (above 40 mg per 100 ml). The degree of impairment of renal function may be shown by (1) the **Creatinine Clearance Test,** which measures the number of millilitres of blood cleared of creatinine per minute (normally about 75 ml); this is a test of glomerular function, and (2) the **Urine Concentration Test,** which gives a measure of tubular function. The patient fasts from after the midday meal and normally one of the specimens passed at 7 a.m., 8 a.m. and 9 a.m. next morning should reach a specific gravity of 1025 or above.

This stage of early chronic renal failure with minimal symptoms may persist for a long time, sometimes years, before the terminal stage is reached.

(*b*) **Terminal Renal Failure (Uraemia).** For convenience the clinical features may be considered systematically:

1 **Central Nervous System.** Increasing tiredness leads eventu-

ally to drowsiness and coma. Muscular twitching and sometimes epileptiform convulsions may occur.

2 **Alimentary System.** The tongue is dry and coated with a dirty brown fur, the breath has a uriniferous odour, and hiccups, nausea and vomiting are common. Haemorrhage into the gut may lead to haematemesis or bloodstained diarrhoea; it is due to mucosal irritation by ammonia derived from the urea excreted by the gut.

3 **Respiratory System.** Failure of the kidneys to eliminate acid leads to its accumulation in the blood and the consequent stimulation of the respiratory centre in the brain causes a gasping type of respiration known as Kussmaul breathing; Cheyne-Stokes respiration may also occur in the terminal stages.

4 **Cardiovascular System** shows effects of the associated high blood pressure: the retina contains haemorrhages and exudates and the left ventricle is hypertrophied. A small proportion of the patients die from heart failure or cerebro-vascular accidents, though the majority die of the renal failure itself. Pericarditis often develops in the final week or two of the illness.

5 **The Skin** is dry and becomes yellowish or brownish in colour; and since the sweat glands eliminate some of the urea and other substances normally excreted by the kidneys generalised irritation (pruritus) is a common symptom.

6 **The Blood** always shows some anaemia.

7 **The Urine** usually has a fixed specific gravity of 1010–1012 and it contains protein and numerous microscopic casts of the renal tubules.

Treatment of Chronic Renal Failure Unfortunately nothing can be done to prevent or delay the fatal outcome in most patients with chronic renal failure and it is important not to increase the patient's discomfort and suffering by therapeutic measures which are of very doubtful value. This observation applies particularly to irksome restrictions in diet. It is true that theoretically protein intake should be reduced when there is severe impairment of renal function (it is recommended that the daily protein should be cut to 40 g when the blood urea rises above 100 mg per 100 ml and to 20 g when the renal failure becomes more severe) and a diet largely composed of carbohydrate and fat should certainly be given, but the time comes when the patient's wishes should receive prior claim over metabolic theory. Many of these patients do not have severe oedema and lose large quantities of sodium in the urine and they may feel better if salt is used in cooking and is taken with meals. Since the kidneys have lost the ability to concentrate, the excretion of urea and other waste products is proportional to the amount of urine passed so that a high urine output is essential and it is important to ensure that the **fluid intake** is at least 3 litres daily.

In the final stages chlorpromazine often prevents nausea and vomiting and morphine may relieve discomfort and alleviate fears and anxiety.

Maintenance Haemodialysis and Renal Transplant It is now possible for some patients in terminal renal failure to be maintained in fair health by haemodialysis; the selection of those who are suitable is a very difficult decision, requiring the evaluation of many medical, psychological and social factors by the renal physician. A permanent arteriovenous communication or fistula is made in the patient's forearm and through this he is attached to a dialysis machine (which may be in his own home) for 12–14 hours two or three times a week. A renal transplant offers another possibility of rescue to the patient in terminal renal failure and if successful enables him to lead a more normal life than is possible for patients on dialysis.

Urinary Tract Infections

Cystitis (inflammation of the bladder) and pyelitis (inflammation of the pelvis of the kidney) are common conditions which result from infection in the urinary tract. At present the word 'pyelo-nephritis' is often used in place of 'pyelitis' to emphasise that there is also inflammation in the substance of the kidney; this point is important, because in patients who have a long history of recurrent or chronic pyelo-nephritis the kidneys may be so damaged that hypertension and renal failure eventually develop. To prevent such serious complications, all urinary tract infections should be treated as promptly and efficiently as possible.

The disease occurs much more often in women, no doubt because the short female urethra gives easier access to the bacteria, and is particularly common in the early weeks of marriage and during pregnancy. Drinking plenty of fluids and emptying the bladder after sexual intercourse often help to prevent recurrent cystitis in young women. Urinary stasis also predisposes to infection, which is frequently seen therefore in men with bladder-neck obstruction due to an enlarged prostate and in patients with a neurological disease such as tabes, which impairs the emptying of the bladder.

Symptoms and Signs The onset is usually sudden, with fever, shivering or rigor, general malaise, aching in one or both loins, and sometimes in the suprapubic region, frequency of micturition and dysuria (painful micturition). There is usually tenderness over one or both kidneys, increase in the white cells in the blood (leucocytosis) and large numbers of pus cells are found on microscopic examination of the urine. *E. coli* is the usual organism isolated when a mid-stream specimen of urine is cultured; less often a streptococcus or *B. proteus* may be found.

Treatment The patient must be nursed in bed while still febrile and persuaded to drink large quantities of bland fluids—at least 3 litres daily. Co-trimoxazole (Septrin) 2 tablets twice daily for 5 days is the antibiotic of choice and usually relieves the symptoms in a day or two; if they persist an unusual organism is probably responsible and the result of the initial urine culture will now reveal what it is. The sensitivity tests done in the laboratory will also show the most suitable antibiotic to use. Patients with chronic or recurrent urinary infection should have a complete urological investigation, including intravenous urography and cystoscopy, so that any stasis or obstruction in the urinary tract may be accurately diagnosed and appropriately treated. A few patients have frequently recurring attacks and may require longer term antibiotic therapy; co-trimoxazole 1 tablet at night or nitrofurantoin 100 mg once or twice daily for up to 6 months are suitable for this purpose.

7
Vitamins

Definition Vitamins are chemical substances whose presence in the diet in adequate amounts is essential for the maintenance of the normal metabolic processes of the body.

Vitamin Deficiency

It follows from the above definition that when the intake of any of the essential vitamins falls below the minimum requirements of the body, symptoms and signs of deficiency will appear. This happens extremely rarely in Britain at the present time, so that primary vitamin deficiency is very uncommon. Certain vitamins, notably vitamin K, folic acid, nicotinic acid and riboflavin, are synthesised by bacteria which normally live in the intestine, and 'conditioned deficiency' of these vitamins may occur if a broad spectrum antibiotic, given for an infection by pathogenic organisms, kills the vitamin-producing bacteria at the same time. For this reason vitamins of the B group are commonly given with broad spectrum antibiotics. Conditioned vitamin deficiency is also seen as a complication of various intestinal disorders which impair the absorption of these essential food factors, or as a result of alcoholism, drug addiction or neglect of a child or elderly person.

Vitamin A

This is one of the fat-soluble vitamins, found in high concentration in fish-liver oils and in eggs, milk and butter. Its precursor (carotene) is present in all coloured fruit and vegetables (including green vegetables); Vitamin A deficiency occurs only when there is insufficient dairy produce, fish and vegetables, and is hardly ever seen except in hot, dry, inland areas in the East.

The signs of deficiency are **night blindness**, dryness and thickening of the conjunctiva (**xerophthalmia**) and **follicular keratosis** (roughening of the skin due to blocking of the follicles with horny plugs).

Vitamin D

This is also a fat-soluble vitamin. Deficiency causes the very important childhood disease, rickets.

Vitamin C (Ascorbic acid)

This is a water-soluble vitamin, and is found in fruit and vegetables. Oranges, lemons, tomatoes, brussels sprouts, black currants and rose-hip extracts are particularly rich sources; potatoes contain less, but nevertheless are the most important antiscorbutic food in this country, in view of the amount eaten.

Deficiency of vitamin C causes **scurvy,** epidemics of which used to occur among sailors on long voyages owing to the lack of fresh vegetables in the diet. It was discovered that orange or lemon juice would prevent such epidemics long before the existence of vitamins was known. Scurvy is very rare in Britain now, though it is still occasionally seen in elderly people who have been living alone in humble circumstances and eating little more than bread and jam for many months. In such patients the scurvy is only one of the more prominent features of the general malnutrition.

Symptoms and Signs of Scurvy The patient is very weak and tired and shows evidence of haemorrhage into the skin, usually in numerous places, either in the form of crops of purpuric spots or as larger areas of bruising (or ecchymoses). Bleeding from various mucous membranes is also common. The most characteristic lesion is seen in the gums, which become spongy and haemorrhagic and show remarkable protrusions ('scurvy buds') a millimetre or so from their junction with the teeth.

Treatment consists in giving a diet rich in foods containing vitamin C, supplemented in the early stages by ascorbic acid 100 mg three times daily.

Vitamin B

This is a water-soluble complex of many different factors, the most important of which are aneurine (or thiamine), nicotinic acid, riboflavin, folic acid and cyanocobalamin (or vitamin B12). It is found mainly in seeds, eggs, the germ and bran of cereals, yeast, meat, fish and milk. Since the various factors of the vitamin B complex occur in the same foods, isolated deficiency of one particular factor is uncommon; there is nearly always multiple deficiency, though in different groups of patients lack of certain factors is relatively more severe.

Beri-beri occurs when there is a predominant deficiency of aneurine (thiamine). It occurs mainly in parts of the East where the staple diet is polished rice (i.e. rice deprived of the pericarp which contains the vitamin), but is very occasionally seen in this country in patients whose diet has been defective as a result of anorexia, food fads or other cause. The patients are not generally undernourished and may, indeed, be quite fat, since beri-beri occurs only when the diet has contained plenty of carbohydrate but insufficient aneurine for the proper metabolism of the carbohydrate. Two forms of the disease are recognised: 'dry' beri-beri, characterised by pains, weakness, wasting and numbness in the legs due to a peripheral neuritis; and 'wet' beri-beri, in which there are massive oedema and other signs of heart failure in addition to the neuritis.

Treatment consists in giving plenty of foods rich in the B complex, substituting wholemeal for white bread and adding yeast or marmite to the diet. At first tablets containing the various B factors may also be prescribed with advantage.

Pellagra is due to predominant deficiency of nicotinic acid and riboflavin, the classical triad of symptoms being diarrhoea, dementia and dermatitis. In fact, however, actual dementia is rare, the commoner neurological manifestations being simply headache, irritability and insomnia. Nausea and vomiting occur almost as often as diarrhoea. The dermatitis is seen mainly on exposed parts, such as the face, the neck and the backs of the hands, and at first looks rather like sunburn, but the affected patches have clearly defined edges and are very persistent, often with a good deal of superficial desquamation. The tongue is often sore, with a red, glazed appearance, and there may be cracking at the angles of the mouth.

Treatment A good mixed diet must be given, with nicotinic acid 100 mg five times daily and riboflavin 1 mg three times daily. The frequently allied deficiency of aneurine and B12 also requires correction.

Vitamin K

This is a fat-soluble vitamin. It is found in certain vegetables and is synthesised by bacterial action in the intestine. Unless there is enough bile in the intestine, it is not absorbed into the blood, and that is why vitamin K deficiency in adults is seen in patients with obstructive jaundice.

The liver requires adequate supplies of vitamin K for the formation of prothrombin, which is one of the substances needed for normal blood-clotting. When vitamin K is deficient, therefore, there is not enough prothrombin in the blood, and persistent bleeding occurs after wounds or injuries because a firm blood-clot fails to form. The deficiency can be corrected by intramuscular injections of vitamin K in doses of 5 mg.

8
The Endocrine System

The endocrine system consists of the ductless glands, which control various functions of the body through the hormones they secrete into the blood. The pituitary gland not only produces hormones which have a direct effect on the body, but also another set of so-called 'trophic' (or nourishing) hormones, which stimulate other endocrine glands to liberate their own hormones. Thus, the pituitary stimulates the thyroid gland by secreting the 'thyrotrophic' hormone, and the adrenal cortex by secreting the 'adrenocorticotrophic hormone' (or ACTH). Furthermore, a delicate balance is maintained between these trophic hormones and the hormones of the glands they stimulate. For example, when an increase in the thyrotrophic hormone from the pituitary stimulates the thyroid to secrete more thyroxin, the increased thyroxin in its turn acts on the pituitary, causing it to reduce the output of thyrotrophic hormone; on the other hand, a reduced output of thyrotrophic hormone leads to a fall in the production of thyroxin and this has the effect of stimulating the pituitary to secrete more thyrotrophic hormone. This mechanism ensures that the concentration of each of these hormones is always kept within the normal physiological range.

The symptoms and signs of diseases affecting the endocrine system are due to the production of either too much or too little hormone by one or more of the ductless glands.

The Thyroid

Thyrotoxicosis

This disease is very much commoner in women than in men and occurs mainly in early adult life. When it does affect older people the clinical features are often less obvious and more easily overlooked.

There is sometimes an abrupt onset of symptoms after an emotional shock which in some unknown way seems to derange the secretion of thyrotrophic hormone by the pituitary. Not only is too much of this hormone produced, thus causing excessive activity of the thyroid, but also the 'switch-off device' described above fails to work, and in spite of the excessive thyroxin produced by the thyroid the pituitary continues to pour out its stimulating thyrotrophic hormone.

Symptoms and Signs With one exception the symptoms and signs are caused by the excessive secretion of thyroxin by the thyroid gland. This hormone controls what is called the metabolic rate; when too much of it is produced the fire of life burns more fiercely and consumes great quantities of fuel. An important symptom therefore is increase in appetite; but even the enormous amounts of food eaten are insufficient to feed the furnace, and the patient's own tissues are consumed. Loss of weight is therefore a prominent feature. The patient usually complains particularly of increased nervousness and excitability, palpitations, sweating, sometimes diarrhoea and occasionally scanty or absent menstrual periods. Since the metabolic 'fire' is using up much more oxygen than normal, the cardiac output of blood is greatly increased to meet the increased demands; for this reason the pulse is rapid, even during sleep. Moreover the 'fire' produces a great deal of heat which the body has to get rid of, so that the skin is always warm and moist.

The one important clinical feature not due to the excess of thyroxin is exophthalmos. This forward protrusion of the eyes, which gives the patient a typical startled expression, is due to the increased output of hormone from the pituitary, and it is therefore the one feature of the disease which often fails to improve following treatment directed to the thyroid gland itself.

Investigation of Thyroid Function The uptake of radio-active iodine by the thyroid gland and the levels of protein-bound iodine, tri-iodothyronine (T3) and thyroxine (T4) in the plasma are all raised in thyrotoxicosis. So is the 'free thyroxine index', obtained by multiplying the T3 resin uptake by the free thyroxine (T4).

In doubtful cases the TSH (thyroid-stimulating hormone) suppression test may be used. Its principle is that if normal subjects are given a thyroid hormone the output of pituitary TSH is greatly reduced, by the switch-off device described above, and thyroid activity as measured by the I131 uptake is greatly reduced; in thyrotoxicosis the switch-off device is not working and the I131 uptake is unchanged.

All tests involving iodine may be vitiated if the patient has recently taken preparations containing iodine (as many cough mixtures do) or has had an injection of iodine-containing contrast medium for an X-ray of the kidneys or gall-bladder (intravenous urogram or cholecystogram).

Treatment Surgical removal of the greater part of the thyroid gland is a satisfactory treatment for most patients. Alternatively a drug may be given which blocks the output of thyroxin from the thyroid. Carbimazole is the drug usually used, in dosage of 20–40 mg daily, gradually reduced over a period of months to 5–10 mg daily. Its disadvantages are that the patient has to be kept under fairly close medical supervision for a long time, since toxic effects of the drug sometimes occur. The most important and dangerous of these is agranulocytosis (reduction or absence of the white blood corpuscles); regular white blood counts are therefore carried out, and the patient is warned that she must stop taking the tablets at once if she develops sore throat, fever or any other unusual symptom. The drug can usually be stopped after nine to twelve months. Therapeutic radio-active iodine is an excellent form of treatment for patients over forty. A beta blocker such as propranolol 20 mg t.d.s. gives rapid relief from the palpitations and feelings of agitation.

Nursing Care A patient with a mild degree of thyrotoxicosis may be treated without coming into hospital, as the environment of a general ward may upset her. There is also an added danger of infection to which these patients are prone.

The severely thyrotoxic patient will, however, require to be in hospital. Rest, both mental and physical, is essential. As this patient always feels hot, she should be in a well-ventilated, airy room with a bed near the window. The bedclothes should be light, and an electric fan may be necessary. It is sometimes advisable for the patient to be in a single room, as she is irritated by noise and easily upset. She is sensitive, excitable, critical, anxious and often very frightened. The nurse must be calm and unruffled at all times and be ready to help her patient through these difficult moods with reassurance and encouragement. The patient may be confined to bed for a short time, but will soon be allowed up for a daily bath and toilet purposes.

The temperature, pulse and respiration will be taken and recorded 4-hourly, the sleeping pulse being the most accurate. Care must be taken to note any irregularity of pulse rhythm, as the toxic state is likely to affect the heart, and atrial fibrillation may occur, in which case it will be necessary to take and record both apex and radial beats. Glycosuria may occur, and the urine should be tested twice weekly.

Sleep is most necessary; when sweating is profuse, sponging with cold water to which a little eau-de-cologne has been added will help to make the patient comfortable and induce sleep. A tranquilliser such as diazepam (Valium) may be ordered. Even during sleep the patient is often restless and suddenly awakens in a frightened state. It is important that any such disturbances should be reported.

The diet should be light, nourishing and of high calorific value. The amount of fluid lost through sweating and attacks of diarrhoea may be considerable, and to replace it at least 2500 ml of fluid should be taken in the 24 hours. This can be given as water, fruit drinks, weak tea and milk drinks.

If exophthalmos is marked, parolene drops should be instilled to protect the cornea and the bed should be in such a position as to avoid direct light.

Response to treatment by carbimazole will be shown by gain in weight, absence of sweating, more normal pulse rate and decrease of nervous tension.

Hypothyroidism

Diminished or absent secretion of thyroxin by the thyroid causes **cretinism** when it is present from birth and **myxoedema** when it comes on in adult life. Only the latter form will be considered here. **Myxoedema** is usually seen in women after the menopause, and the clinical effects are due to the metabolic 'fire' burning abnormally low. The patient therefore becomes mentally and physically sluggish, feels weak and tired, loses her appetite, puts on weight, becomes very sensitive to cold and complains of constipation. The face has a puffy, dull, expressionless appearance, usually showing a general waxy pallor with sometimes a little patch of colour on each cheek (the 'malar flush'). The skin is cold, rough and dry, and the hair thin, coarse and lifeless. The voice often develops a typical hoarse monotonous quality and the patient speaks slowly and infrequently. The pulse-rate is slow. There is always some anaemia. In advanced cases either heart failure or severe mental changes may occur. The I131 uptake and the levels of protein-bound iodine, T3 and T4 in the plasma, and the 'free thyroxine index' are all reduced (see 'investigation of thyroid function', p. 118).

Treatment consists in giving tablets of sodium l-thyroxine. Initial large doses may be dangerous, and it is usual to start with not more than 0.1 mg daily, slowly increasing to three to five times this amount, according to the clinical response. Treatment must of course be continued regularly for the rest of the patient's life.

The Adrenal Glands

The two adrenal glands each consist of a cortex and a medulla. The function of these two parts of the glands is quite distinct, and only the cortex will be considered in this section.

Three main groups of hormones are produced by the adrenal cortex:

1 The sugar-regulating hormone, whose action is similar to the synthetic cortisone; excess causes conversion of body protein into sugar and raises the blood-sugar level.

2 The salt-regulating hormone, aldosterone; excess causes loss of potassium and retention in the body of sodium, which holds with it an osmotically equivalent volume of water, and so may lead to oedema.

3 Sex hormones, mainly androgens which in excess cause the development of male secondary sex characteristics in women.

Cushing's Syndrome

This syndrome is due to excessive production of adrenal cortical hormones, either by a tumour, or by generalised hyperplasia (overgrowth) of the adrenal cortex, or by excessive stimulation of it by increased output of ACTH (adrenocorticotrophic hormone) from the pituitary. The striking clinical features are great obesity, confined to the face and trunk; in women hair grows on the face and chest and the periods usually stop; broad purple lines appear over the abdomen, thighs and buttocks from weakening and rupture of the deeper layers of the skin, which also becomes coarse and rough; the blood-sugar may be raised; the spine may become kyphotic (bent forward) from loss of protein from the bone.

Treatment An operation is carried out to remove the adrenal tumour or the greater part of the adrenal cortex on both sides.

Addison's Disease

This disease is due to lack of the adrenal cortical hormones, and results from complete destruction of the adrenal cortex on both sides by either tuberculosis or simple atrophy. The clinical features are great weakness, loss of weight, indigestion, low blood pressure, attacks of faintness due to low blood-sugar (hypoglycaemia) and pigmentation, which causes brownish discoloration most obvious on the exposed areas of skin, such as the face, neck and arms, and is sometimes seen also in the mucous membrane of the mouth.

The pigmentation is now thought to be due to over-action of the pigmentary hormone of the pituitary, which is normally balanced and checked by a hormone from the adrenal cortex. The **Addisonian Crisis** is a medical emergency of great importance, since the patient will almost certainly die within two or three days if it is not treated promptly and skilfully. It is heralded by severe vomiting, which quickly leads to dehydration and collapse, and the systolic blood pressure may fall to 50 or even lower. Patients with Addison's disease may be precipitated into crisis by any intercurrent infection, accident or shock or by certain drugs such as morphine or insulin.

Treatment Most patients do best on a combination of cortisone 12.5–25 mg twice daily and fluorocortisone 0.2 mg once or twice daily. They should carry a card stating the diagnosis; details of their maintenance therapy; and instructions to double or treble the dosage should unusual stress occur. Patients in crisis require large amounts of intravenous fluid and cortisone, starting with normal saline containing 100 mg hydrocortisone in 500 ml.

The Anterior Lobe of the Pituitary

Gigantism and **Acromegaly** are due to excessive production of the growth hormone by a tumour of certain cells in the anterior lobe of the pituitary. In children or adolescents it produces a generalised abnormal increase in growth known as gigantism; in adults whose epiphyses have united, and whose long bones are unable therefore to increase in length, it produces acromegaly (literally, 'enlargement of the extremities'). The hands, feet and lower jaw become enormous, the skin and subcutaneous tissues are thickened, and there is enlargement too of the internal organs. Pressure from the tumour in the pituitary causes severe headache and sometimes restriction of the temporal fields of vision. Deep X-ray therapy to the pituitary is the usual treatment.

Simmond's Disease is due to destruction of the anterior lobe of the pituitary, usually by an infarct occurring during the period of shock following a severe postpartum haemorrhage. The first symptom is often failure of lactation, the menstrual periods fail to return, the patient becomes weak and tired and loses interest in life, the axillary and pubic hair are gradually lost and the skin shows striking lack of pigmentation. Treatment is always difficult and often unsatisfactory; a combination of testosterone, cortisone and l-thyroxine may be given, but great caution has to be observed, since alarming reactions to even small doses of one or other of these preparations are not uncommon.

The Posterior Lobe of the Pituitary

Diabetes Insipidus is due to lack of the antidiuretic hormone of the posterior lobe of the pituitary. This hormone normally controls re-absorption of water by the renal tubules; in its absence the kidneys secrete enormous quantities of very dilute urine, which contains neither sugar nor albumin. The principal symptom is the thirst which results from the consequent dehydration.

Treatment The symptoms can usually be controlled by posterior pituitary extract taken in the form of snuff.

Diabetes Mellitus

This common and important disease can be roughly subdivided into two main clinical varieties:

1 acute severe diabetes occurring in thin young people, and
2 a milder form affecting middle-aged or elderly people who are overweight.

This classification is important, since the two groups of patients require different treatment. The first variety is due to failure of the pancreas to produce enough insulin, and injections of insulin are necessary for its control; the second variety is due in some obscure way to overloading of the body with fat, and as there is no shortage of insulin the appropriate treatment is not insulin injections but weight reduction.

Symptoms and Signs In both clinical types the metabolic upset causes the blood-sugar to be abnormally high (hyperglycaemia) and in consequence sugar 'spills over' into the urine. The glucose passing down the renal tubules holds with it an osmotically equivalent volume of water, so that the primary symptom is **polyuria** (passage of excessive amounts of urine). This loss of water causes dehydration, so that the second main symptom is **thirst.** The wastage of sugar leads to **tiredness, loss of weight** and sometimes more remote effects such as **amenorrhoea. Pruritus** (itching) of the vulva is common, no doubt because the sugar in the urine encourages infection.

The urine contains large amounts of sugar, and in the acute variety of the disease acetone bodies also.

Diagnosis In patients presenting the above clinical picture the diagnosis is obvious, but sometimes routine examination reveals sugar in the urine of a patient who has no symptoms, and then a **glucose tolerance test** has to be done to find out if he has diabetes or simply a harmless type of glycosuria. The patient is given no breakfast, and at the start of the test he empties his bladder and has a specimen of blood taken for estimation of his fasting blood-sugar level. He is then given a drink containing 50 g of glucose, and samples of blood and urine are taken every ½ hour for the next 3 hours. Patients with diabetes have an abnormally high fasting blood sugar, and after taking the sugar it rises even higher throughout the whole period of the test. Sugar is also found in the specimens of urine. In the harmless varieties of glycosuria it is found either that the urine contains sugar though the blood sugar is never abnormally high, or that the blood sugar rises to a high level and spills over into the urine for ½–1 hour after the glucose has been drunk but quickly falls to a normal level again well before the end of the test.

Complications are very numerous and may affect every system of the body.

Diabetic Coma is the most dangerous of them, and must always be treated as an acute medical emergency. The complication is particularly to be feared in the acute diabetes of thin young people; fat diabetics rarely if ever develop ketosis, which is the main cause of the coma. The ketone bodies (exemplified by the acetone which can be detected in the breath and urine) are normal end-products of the metabolism of fat; in diabetic coma excessive quantities of them have been formed because the severe upset in carbohydrate metabolism has forced the body to use fat as its principal source of energy. A dangerous degree of ketosis therefore occurs only when the utilisation of sugar by the body is severely curtailed, either because the patient for some reason has failed to take his insulin, or because an intercurrent infection has temporarily increased his insulin requirements.

Non-ketotic (Hyperosmolar) Coma is a complication seen particularly in elderly obese diabetics. It is more common in women, and in the UK is seen mainly in West Indian immigrants. The clinical features are mental confusion or coma, dehydration, a very high blood-sugar level and absence of ketosis. Treatment is insulin and IV 0.5 normal saline.

When a patient under treatment for diabetes lapses into coma, the question calling for immediate answer is whether it is diabetic coma or insulin coma. Insulin coma results when too big a dose has been given, or when the normal dose has not been followed by the normal breakfast, the loss of consciousness being due to the profound fall in the blood-sugar level (hypoglycaemia). Fortunately the distinction can usually be made without great difficulty. As explained above, diabetic coma occurs only in patients whose diabetic state has been badly out of control, and relatives or friends will usually say that the patient has not been well for a few days, feeling tired, having polyuria, thirst, headache, constipation and abdominal pain. He may also show evidence of a boil, carbuncle or other infection which has temporarily increased the severity of his diabetes. By contrast, the patient in insulin coma has been perfectly well until the injection of insulin an hour or two previously, and before losing consciousness he has complained of symptoms of hypoglycaemia: an empty sinking feeling in the epigastrium, faintness, sweating, palpitations and unsteadiness. The patient in diabetic coma is grossly dehydrated, having a dry tongue, soft eyeballs and lax, inelastic skin, and large amounts of acetone are present in his breath and urine. The hypoglycaemic patient is neither dehydrated nor ketotic. In diabetic coma the urine is loaded with sugar; in hypoglycaemic coma there is no sugar in the urine unless the bladder happens to contain urine secreted an hour or two earlier, and then there is not usually more than a trace. The blood sugar is very high in diabetic coma and very low in insulin coma, but the diagnosis has to be made and treatment started before the result of this estimation is known.

Diabetic gangrene of the feet is a serious complication in middle-aged and elderly patients. It is due partly to reduction in the blood supply from atheroma in the arteries, and partly to infection. For reasons not fully understood, severe atheroma is common in diabetics, and their tissues generally are very prone to infections.

Skin infections, particularly boils and carbuncles, are common.

Pulmonary tuberculosis is another infection which diabetics acquire more often than other people, and before the days of insulin it was a common cause of death.

Cataract, peripheral neuritis (causing pains, tingling, numbness and weakness in the legs), and a special type of **nephritis** (revealed by heavy albuminuria) are other important diabetic complications.

Treatment Weight reduction is usually all that is necessary for a fat patient with relatively mild diabetes. He should be given a low-calorie diet severely restricted in both carbohydrate and fat and instructed to weigh himself weekly on reliable scales, always in the same clothes and at the same time of the day. He should also be told that if he has not lost at least a pound the first week he must take smaller helpings next week and continue this depressing process until he does lose weight. This manoeuvre puts the onus on the patient and prevents his returning in a month, fatter than ever, and saying complacently, 'I took your diet and look at me now'. Fat patients who do succeed in reducing to near their normal weight usually lose all clinical evidence of the diabetic state, as well as sparing themselves from various other serious complications of obesity, so that their self-denial is well worth while.

Some late-onset mild diabetics are not adequately controlled by diet alone and may be improved by oral glibenclamide, tolbutamide or chlorpropamide. All other diabetics require treatment with both diet and insulin.

In constructing a diabetic diet it has been traditional to keep the amount of carbohydrate low (usually 150–200 g daily for an adult), to prescribe about 70 g protein daily and to make up the balance of calories with fat. Recently, however, such diets have been criticised on the grounds that large amounts of animal fat are likely to increase the already high risk to diabetics of arterial complications. The present tendency, therefore, is to prescribe a diet low in animal fat, and with a high-fibre high carbohydrate content (but excluding sugar).

Insulin was formerly available in three strengths, 20 units per ml, 40 units per ml and 80 units per ml (injected by a syringe graduated in 20 divisions to the ml) but from 1st March 1983 all diabetics have been changed to the new single strength insulin. This is U100 insulin containing 100 units per ml (injected by a new U100 syringe graduated in 100 units to the ml) (see Figure facing). It is hoped this change will eliminate confusion and make it easier for diabetics to be sure they are giving themselves the correct dose.

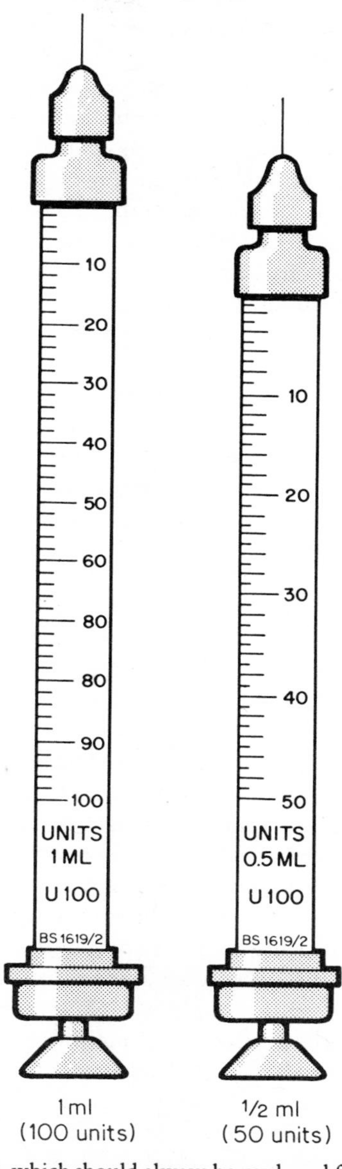

1 ml
(100 units)

1/2 ml
(50 units)

U 100 diabetic syringes, which should always be used used for giving U 100 insulin (courtesy of Mrs P. John)

Soluble insulin is quickly absorbed into the blood, so that its effect is greatest in about 2–3 hours and over in about 6 hours. Patients having soluble insulin therefore have to be given at least two injections daily, usually 20 minutes before breakfast and 20 minutes before the evening meal. Other 'depot' preparations release the insulin more slowly over a longer period, and many patients can be kept under satisfactory control throughout the 24 hours with one injection daily. Protamine zinc insulin (PZI) and insulin zinc suspension lente (IZS) are the two depot insulins in most common use. Some patients develop allergic reactions to their insulin injections and should be changed to the more purified so-called monocomponent insulins (e.g. Actrapid MC, whose activity lasts 2–4 hours and Rapidard MC, with an activity lasting 4–10 hours). These insulins should also be used in pregnancy since antibodies induced by impure insulins may damage the foetal islet cells.

Nursing Care From the moment the patient comes into hospital for stabilisation it is important to help him to adopt the right attitude towards his condition, namely that he is going to be able to keep well and lead a fully active life as long as he makes certain adjustments in his diet and takes insulin.

To help the patient achieve this a simple explanation of the cause of the condition and the effect of insulin therapy should be given. In addition, the patient must have adequate instruction in the technique of giving insulin, and factors which might interfere with its effect should be discussed.

During stabilisation he should be kept active so that his calorie requirements and insulin dosage can be calculated on much the same amount of energy as he expends in his normal life.

It is the nurse's responsibility to see that the patient realises the importance of keeping to the diet and not eating anything his friends and relations may bring in when visiting him. Meals must be given at the correct time and a note made of any food left, as adjustment in the amount of insulin given may be necessary. She must give the patient a simple understanding of food values, particularly of carbohydrates, and explain the way in which he can vary his diet according to his tastes. Emphasis should be put on his taking as normal a diet as possible, so that it does not become a burden to himself and other people. Before leaving hospital he will be given diet sheets showing alternative foods with approximate calorific values. His weight will be checked twice weekly at first and later at longer intervals.

Insulin has to be given by subcutaneous injection, and the great majority of diabetics, even children, quickly learn how to do this for themselves. In the early stages of treatment, therefore, the nurse must instruct the patient in the handling and sterilising of the syringe and in giving the injections, showing the various sites which can be used in rotation to prevent soreness of one area. When patients are elderly or the sight is poor an intelligent relative may be willing to learn to do it for them, or, failing this, a District Nurse is asked to call on the patient.

Patients being stabilised on insulin are given a suitable diet, and their urine is tested every 4 hours for sugar and acetone. The findings are recorded on a special chart, together with the amount of insulin given. Blood sugar estimations can now be performed by many patients at home and give a much more accurate picture of the control of the diabetes than urine tests. All patients must be taught how to test either the blood or urine, must be urged to perform these tests regularly and must be given a clear but simple explanation of the significance of the results. Some patients are difficult to stabilise, and the nurse must be aware of the signs of insulin overdosage, namely, hunger, faintness, palpitations, sweating, unsteadiness and drowsiness, which if not treated promptly will progress to coma. A drink containing 30 g glucose (1 oz) must be given to prevent this occurring. The patient himself must at some stage be taught to recognise the symptoms of hypoglycaemia by being given a deliberate overdose of insulin so that in future he will know the danger signals and how to avert actual coma. Every diabetic taking insulin should carry a few lumps of sugar with him for this purpose. He should in addition carry with him at all times a card and preferably also wear either a medallion or bracelet stating that he is a diabetic and giving the name of the doctor who is treating him and his dosage of insulin.

General Health Diabetes is affected by the general health of the patient, and he should be taught to look after himself very carefully. Diabetics, particularly those of middle age and beyond, suffer from poor circulation. Healing power and resistance to infection are poor, and they should therefore be instructed to take particular care of the feet, because even a minor infection may be an important factor in the development of gangrene. The feet should be washed daily, carefully dried and powdered and clean socks put on. The toenails should be cut frequently and with care, so that any in-growing tendency is prevented, and fungus or other infections must receive immediate and thorough treatment. Good footwear is most important, in order to prevent any friction or pressure. Corns and callouses may give rise to much trouble; they should not be treated by the patient or his friends, but by a chiropodist who has been informed of the patient's condition. The skin must be kept very clean and good oral hygiene is important; regular visits should be made to the dentist.

While the patient is in hospital the nurse must make sure that he has a daily bath (which must not be too hot), that he learns to look after himself satisfactorily and that he understands the reason for so doing. Special attention must be given to any septic spots or boils. The patient is taught how to avoid as far as possible such infections as colds, sore throats, influenza. If infection or illness of any kind occurs he must realise that stabilisation is likely to be upset and that he must consult his doctor at once.

Treatment of Diabetic Coma Admission to hospital as a medical emergency is essential. A large dose of soluble insulin, 50–100 units, is given at once and an intravenous infusion of normal saline set up, the first 2 litres being run in quickly. If the patient is still in deep coma 2 hours later another 50 units of insulin are given, and the need for subsequent doses is decided on the result of blood-sugar estimations. Usually some 200–300 units, or even more, are required in the first 24 hours, and it is nearly always necessary to continue the intravenous saline at a slower rate of administration throughout the first day. Estimation of the blood electrolytes may reveal other disturbances which require correction; in particular, it is often advisable to give potassium chloride 1 g four-hourly for a few doses as soon as the patient can swallow. Search should also be made for the infection which may have precipitated the coma and any necessary treatment given.

Treatment of Hypoglycaemic (Insulin) Coma Intravenous injection of 10–20 ml of a sterile solution of 50 per cent glucose leads to immediate recovery of consciousness. If the patient is still able to swallow, it is simpler and better to give sugar by mouth; if he cannot swallow and a suitable solution for intravenous injection is not available, 50 g of sugar in a few ounces of water should be given through a stomach tube. Alternatively, an intramuscular injection of glucagon 1–2 mg will raise his blood-sugar level and may bring him round sufficiently to enable him to swallow.

9

The Chronic Rheumatic Diseases and the Collagen Diseases

Rheumatoid Arthritis

Arthritis means inflammation of a joint. Rheumatoid arthritis is a particular variety characterised by chronic inflammation and eventual deformity in many joints throughout the body. Its cause is unknown. It is several times commoner in women than in men, and usually starts sometime between early adult life and middle age. The disease may be precipitated or aggravated by worry, emotional shocks, overwork or exposure to cold and damp.

Clinical Features Although the local changes in various joints are its most prominent feature, rheumatoid arthritis is a generalised disease of the body which runs a course over many years. During this time there are phases when the disease becomes more active, characterised by fever, anaemia, increase in the white cells in the blood (leucocytosis), a very high sedimentation rate and feelings of exhaustion and general malaise; and quiescent phases when the patient feels much better. Eventually the disease may 'burn itself out': the temperature, blood count, sedimentation rate and general well-being return to normal, but the patient is left with a variable amount of permanent disability, according to the extent of the damage done to the affected joints.

The small joints of the fingers and toes are usually the first to be involved by rheumatoid arthritis, but later the wrists, elbows, shoulders, knees, ankles and temperomandibular joints are frequently affected. These joints become painful, stiff and swollen, and the muscles surrounding them become strikingly wasted. In the later stages the combination of muscular spasm and weakness tends to cause certain deformities: the most characteristic of these is ulnar deviation of the fingers, which, together with the spindle-shaped swelling of the proximal interphalangeal and metacarpophalangeal joints and the muscular atrophy, gives a very typical appearance to the hands in chronic rheumatoid arthritis.

Treatment and Nursing Care During the acute stage care is directed towards prevention of deformities and contractures and the relief of pain. The joints are inflamed and therefore, as with any inflamed part, rest is essential. Rest in bed may have to be continued for many weeks or even months until a remission occurs.

Bed and Position A firm mattress ensures support for the affected parts, and the weight of the bedclothes must be taken by use of a cradle. The position depends on which parts are affected, but shoulders are often painful, and the patient will be most comfortable if sitting up with the arms supported by pillows. To prevent fixed flexion of the hip joints the patient should lie flat for an hour twice a day. Inflamed knee-joints are more comfortable bent than straight, but must on no account be allowed to become fixed in this position. They must be kept straight by use of light splints to prevent deformity which would interfere with walking. A pillow should not be placed under the knee. Support for the feet may be given by a foot-board suitably placed, or by a light plaster or plastic splint.

The wrist and fingers are most commonly affected. The wrist tends to bend downwards and the fingers towards the little finger (ulnar deviation). This particular deformity leaves the hand very weak, and steps should be taken to prevent it by supporting the hands, if necessary by splinting, with the wrists dorsiflexed and the fingers slightly flexed.

To prevent joint fixation full passive movement of affected joints must be performed at least twice daily, and muscle wasting is minimised by insisting on isometric contractions of surrounding muscles at least 12 times every hour. In both acute and subacute stages much improvement may result from the local injection of 50–100 mg hydrocortisone into the affected joint. In the chronic phase orthopaedic and manipulative procedures including synovectomy may be of value.

General Care During the active phase the temperature is often raised, but even if it is normal the patient tends to sweat, particularly in the axillae and groins, back of the neck and palms of the hands. Daily bathing is essential to keep the patient clean and fresh, and a little eau-de-Cologne added to the water will help to counteract the rather sour smell associated with the sweating. While washing the patient, the nurse must be careful to support the limbs by placing her hands under them, and wash them from above downwards, as this helps to prevent the flexion deformities. All splints are removed for washing, and as the pain subsides passive movements may be given at this time. Later active movements will be encouraged.

Diet To help in building up the patient's general health she must receive a varied and well-balanced diet. The fluid intake should be increased during the acute phases. The appetite must be tempted, as the patient will often feel exhausted and unable to make the effort to take her meals. Every encouragement must be given, and if the temporomandibular joint is affected special soft foods will be provided.

For the correction of anaemia, iron is given either by mouth, intramuscularly or intravenously (for details see p. 33); but frequently a small blood transfusion gives better results, and apart from raising the haemoglobin level, seems to have a general beneficial effect on the course of the disease.

Relief of Pain Simple application of heat, such as warm wool and light kaolin poultices, can be very beneficial. Other forms of heat, such as infrared, short-wave diathermy or wax baths, may be ordered, the object being to improve the blood supply to the joints and to relax the tight muscles so that more movement is possible. Aspirin given before nursing treatments will facilitate movement and the patient will be less upset. Aspirin and applications of heat should be given before physiotherapy. To ensure a night's sleep 1–2 tablets of nitrazepam (Mogadon) may be prescribed.

Bowels and Bladder Careful positioning and padding of the bed-pan are necessary because of the discomfort which may be experienced by sitting on it. The patient may try to avoid this, and so become constipated, so that a mild aperient is often necessary. A female urinal or kidney shaped dish may be used when nursing women patients.

Specific Measures

1 **Salicylates** are analgesic and in large doses anti-inflammatory. Soluble aspirin 4–6 g every 24 hours is usually satisfactory but should not be given to patients with peptic ulcers.

2 Other anti-inflammatory analgesics include **indomethacin** 25 mg three times daily or as a 100 mg suppository at night (side-effects: headache or, rarely, mental confusion) and **piroxicam** (Feldene) 20 mg daily, which is also very effective but also occasionally causes serious side-effects.

3 **Steroid Hormones** are effective in relieving symptoms, but

their withdrawal is usually followed by relapse and their long-continued use causes many serious side-effects. They are best given in short courses with gold.

4 **Gold.** Some physicians try the effect of a course of gold injections on patients whose disease remains active after a reasonable period of conservative management. A test dose of 10 mg is given first and the total dosage should not exceed 1 g, divided into 20 injections of 50 mg each given at weekly intervals. Toxic effects include skin rashes, blood disorders and renal damage. Before each injection inquiry is made about irritation at the site of the last injection (and if present no further injections are given); the urine is tested for protein before each injection; and frequent blood counts are taken.

5 **Penicillamine** has recently been shown to be effective in reducing the activity of rheumatoid disease. It is given by mouth, starting with one 250 mg capsule daily and increasing the daily dose by 250 mg every two weeks to a maximum dose of 6 capsules daily. This slowly increasing dosage is thought to reduce the incidence of side-effects, which include skin rashes, sickness, kidney damage and blood disorders; for early detection of the last two, regular urine testing and blood counts are essential.

It should be remembered that the patient is only in hospital in the acute stage and must learn to live with the disease for the rest of her life. Treatment at home will be guided by her own doctor and physiotherapist, but a great deal depends on the patient herself. Perseverance and will-power can do a great deal to prevent invalidism, and relatives and friends should realise that the more the patient is able to do for herself the better. If deformity is crippling, many helpful appliances are available which will render her more independent. Recreational therapy may be of value, but whenever possible the patient should continue to work.

Osteo-arthritis

Osteo-arthritis differs from rheumatoid arthritis in being a purely local disease of the affected joints unaccompanied by any disturbance in the general health of the patient. The change in the joints can be regarded as due to 'wear and tear': consequently they occur only in people of middle age or beyond, they mainly affect weight-bearing joints such as those of the spine and the hips and the knees, and they are aggravated by anything which puts an added strain on the joints, such as obesity or abnormal posture.

Women shortly after the menopause sometimes develop a special variety of osteo-arthritis characterised by the appearance of small bumps known as Heberden's nodes at the terminal interphalangeal joints of the fingers. This variety usually runs a limited course over a matter of months and the prognosis is good.

In the commoner type of degenerative osteo-arthritis, which, as already explained, is due to partial wearing-out of the affected joints, recovery cannot of course be expected, and treatment has to be directed first to relieving the pain and stiffness of which the patient complains, and secondly to reducing the strain on the joints and so slowing down the process of further degeneration. The simplest and best way to relieve the symptoms is to give aspirin 600 mg three or four times daily; physiotherapy, particularly radiant heat or short-wave therapy, is also temporarily soothing, but in the long run is usually less effective than aspirin and it is certainly more time-consuming and expensive. To ease the strain on the joints an attempt should always be made to reduce obesity by dieting, and abnormal postures should be corrected if possible. Severe pain sometimes continues in spite of these measures, particularly in elderly patients with osteo-arthritis of the hip or knee, and surgical arthrodesis of the affected joint may have to be performed.

The Collagen Diseases

This term is used for a group of diseases in which changes in connective tissue are thought to be the main cause of symptoms and signs. In addition to Rheumatic fever and Rheumatoid arthritis the group includes Systemic Lupus Erythematosus (SLE) and Polyarteritis Nodosa (PAN).

Systemic Lupus Erythematosus

This is a disease of young women. Fever, anaemia and leucopenia are usual and in addition many patients have arthritis similar to rheumatoid arthritis and skin rashes, particularly on the face. Other organs sometimes involved are the liver, with resultant jaundice; the heart, leading occasionally to heart failure; and the kidneys, shown first by proteinuria and often later by the nephrotic syndrome and renal failure. The diagnosis is confirmed by finding typical LE cells in the blood; these are leucocytes containing ingested dead nuclear material. Many patients die within a few years but the prognosis is improved by steroid therapy, usually with prednisolone.

Polyarteritis Nodosa

This disease is characterised by fever, loss of weight, tachycardia, very high ESR and anaemia with leucocytosis and eosinophilia. Apart from these common features, the patients can be divided into two clinical types:

1 *With lung involvement.* This type has an equal sex incidence and occurs at any age. It presents with asthma, chronic bronchitis and recurrent pneumonia; the eosinophil count is always very high; there are sometimes granulomatous lesions in the nose.

2 *Without lung involvement.* This type is twice as common in men and the incidence increases with age. Clinical features include abdominal pain, sometimes actual ulcerative colitis, nephritis, peripheral neuritis, arthritis of rheumatoid type and coronary thrombosis.

The diagnosis may be confirmed by biopsy of a pectoral muscle. Ninety per cent of patients are dead within 5 years.

Ankylosing Spondylitis

This is a disease of unknown cause which is at least ten times commoner in men than in women and mainly occurs in young adults. The first symptom is usually pain and stiffness in the back and, as the name implies, the whole spine may eventually become united into one continuous piece of bone by ankylosis of the intervertebral joints. Limitation of movement in the spine is therefore an important physical sign, and it will usually be seen too that the normal lumbar lordosis has been lost and that there is some flexion of the cervical spine. Ankylosis of the joints between the ribs and the vertebrae also occurs and in consequence expansion of the chest becomes painful and limited; for this reason sudden movements such as a sneeze may cause excruciating pain in the thorax. The radiological appearances are typical, particularly in the sacro-iliac joints, and the sedimentation rate is usually very high.

Treatment The aim is to relieve pain and stiffness by giving a non-steroidal anti-inflammatory drug, thus permitting the patient to take part in the vigorous physiotherapy necessary to restore and maintain spinal mobility and prevent flexion deformity of the spine. Indomethacin 25 mg t.d.s. is often very effective for this purpose. The patient should lie prone as much as possible and practise mobilising exercises daily for the rest of his life.

Gout

Gout is a hereditary disease and well over half the patients know of other cases in the family, usually including the father or grandfather. Nearly all the patients are men, and it is uncommon under the age of 40.

The first attack of acute gout usually starts with severe pain and tenderness in the metatarsophalangeal joint of the big toe, which becomes very swollen, red and shiny. After a few days the inflammation subsides and the patient remains perfectly well perhaps for many months until another similar attack of acute arthritis occurs either in the same joint or elsewhere. Through the years after a long succession of attacks there is a tendency for residual permanent changes to occur in the affected joints and the patient has now entered the stage of chronic gout. One of the prominent features of the disease now is the appearance of deposits of sodium biurate (known as 'tophi') round the joints, in the cartilage of the ears and in the olecranon bursae at the elbows. These tophi sometimes ulcerate through the skin and discharge a chalky-white substance.

The diagnosis is confirmed by the radiological appearance of the joints and by the finding of a raised blood uric-acid level.

Treatment Acute gout usually responds satisfactorily to colchicine, which is given by mouth in a dosage of 0.5 mg every 2 hours until symptoms are relieved. Unfortunately colchicine also causes toxic effects, particularly diarrhoea and vomiting, and has been largely superseded by phenylbutazone 100 mg three times daily.

During the acute attack the patient should be nursed in bed with the affected joint protected by a cradle and soothed by the application of cold compresses. He should be given a light diet with plenty of fluids. Until the colchicine takes effect analgesics such as aspirin 0.65 g or even pethidine 50 mg will be required to relieve the pain.

Patients with a tendency to gout should be advised to avoid

articles of food rich in purines, that is to say foods whose metabolism leads to the formation of uric acid. The forbidden foods include liver, kidney, sweet-breads, heart, herring, sardines and fish-roe. Beer and heavy wines such as port and sherry should also be avoided. The elimination of uric acid from the body is increased by probenecid, or allopurinol may be given to limit the production of uric acid in the body.

Lumbago and Sciatica

Lumbago means pain in the lumbar region of the back and **sciatica** is pain in the distribution of the sciatic nerve in the leg. Each of them may be due to any one of a number of different causes; they frequently occur together because a disease affecting the lumbar spine and causing lumbago may also press on the emerging roots of the sciatic nerve and cause sciatica.

By far the commonest cause of lumbago is a tear in the capsule of a lumbar intervertebral disc; if part of the soft central part of the disc is squeezed out through the hole in the capsule and presses on a nerve-root the patient develops sciatica as well. Note that the disc itself is not displaced, so that the expression 'slipped disc' is wrong and should never be used; it gives the patient a quite erroneous idea of what has happened and causes unnecessary anxiety.

Before starting treatment it is wise to exclude the rarer and more serious causes of lumbago and sciatica, particularly secondary carcinoma and tuberculosis of the spine, by having an X-ray taken and estimating the blood sedimentation rate.

Treatment of Lumbar Disc Lesions Since it is flexion of the spine which tends to cause protrusion of the central pulpy nucleus through the tear in the disc capsule, the main object of treatment is to maintain the spine in the erect or extended position until healing has occurred. This may be done either by keeping the patient flat in bed for four to six weeks, preferably using fracture boards and certainly not allowing him to sit up; or by applying a plaster or other form of spinal support which prevents flexion of the lumbar spine. When sciatica is very persistent carefully controlled spinal traction may help to relieve pressure on the affected nerve-root and short-wave therapy may be soothing. In very severe and chronic cases operation may eventually be needed to remove the prolapsed part of the damaged disc.

10

The Nervous System

Anatomy and Physiology

The nervous system comprises the brain and the spinal cord, which together form the central nervous system (CNS), the peripheral nervous system (or peripheral nerves) and the autonomic nervous system. The brain includes the two cerebral hemispheres, the cerebellum and the brain-stem, which is made up of the mid-brain, the pons and the medulla.

The delicate tissues of the brain and spinal cord are protected from injury firstly by being enclosed within the bony walls of the skull and vertebral column, and secondly by the 'cushion' of cerebrospinal fluid in which they float. Three membranes surround the brain and spinal cord: the outermost and toughest is the dura, the middle one is the arachnoid and the innermost and most delicate is the pia. The cerebrospinal fluid (CSF) lies between the arachnoid and the pia in what is known as the subarachnoid space. It is manufactured by the choroid plexuses, which are specialised structures lying inside the cavities (known as ventricles) within the brain; from here the fluid passes out into the subarachnoid space, which surrounds the whole of the brain and spinal cord; and finally it is re-absorbed into the blood by other specialised structures called arachnoid villi, which lie in the venous sinuses.

The nervous system provides one of the main means whereby the activities of the body are regulated in accordance with its needs. To this end the system is made up of millions of neurones, each of which consists of a nerve-cell and its processes or nerve-fibres, and these neurones are grouped into various pathways along which impulses travel from one part of the body to another. By this arrangement an event in one part is signalled to another, which reacts appropriately. The system involves a chain of neurones, the first (or 'receptor') being concerned with reporting or receiving the information, the last (or 'effector') with promoting the appropriate reaction, while interspersed between may be a variable number of linkage (or 'connector') neurones which introduce the possibility of alternative pathways and so variety of response. This chain of neurones which establishes the link between cause and effect is the functional unit of the nervous system and is called the **reflex arc.** By long-established clinical usage the receptor pathways of the reflex arc are referred to as 'sensory neurones' and the effector pathways as 'motor neurones'.

The Motor Neurones are subdivided into the upper motor neurones and the lower motor neurones (see Figure on p. 142). The cells of the upper motor neurones lie in the motor areas of the cortex of the two cerebral hemispheres; the fibres from these cells collect together in a part of the base of each hemisphere known as the internal capsule, run down the brain-stem as far as the medulla, where they cross to the opposite side and then run down in the lateral column of the spinal cord to end by uniting with the nerve-cells of the lower motor neurones. These lie in the anterior part of the spinal cord on each side (hence their alternative name 'anterior horn cells'); their nerve-fibres pass out in the anterior nerve-roots to be distributed by the peripheral nerves to all the voluntary muscles of the body. Before any movement conceived in the brain can be carried out a message has to travel from the cortex all the way down the upper motor neurone to the anterior horn cell, and then along the lower motor neurone to the muscle.

Such a message may be interrupted in its course along the upper motor neurone or along the lower motor neurone; in other words, paralysis or paresis (that is, partial paralysis) of voluntary movement may be due to an upper motor neurone lesion or a lower motor neurone lesion.

Signs of an Upper Motor Neurone Lesion

1 The affected limbs are weak, the degree of weakness varying from patient to patient according to the extent of the upper motor neurone lesion.

2 The weak limbs are spastic: that is, they are in spasm or have increased muscular tone; and since the briskness of the tendon reflexes is accentuated when the muscles have increased tone, the tendon jerks are exaggerated.

3 The weak muscles do not undergo wasting, except to a very slight extent as a result of disuse.

4 When the sole of the foot is firmly stroked with a blunt object the big toe turns upwards instead of downwards; in other words, the plantar response becomes extensor instead of flexor.

Signs of a Lower Motor Neurone Lesion

1 The affected muscles again show a variable degree of weakness, from complete paralysis to slight paresis.

2 The muscles become very strikingly wasted. This muscular atrophy is the most prominent feature of lower motor neurone lesions; it is due to the fact that in health the lower motor neurone is necessary for maintaining the tone and nutrition of the muscles.

3 For this reason, loss of the lower motor neurone results in loss of muscular tone and flaccidity of the limb and this in turn causes

4 Weakness or absence of the tendon reflexes. The plantar reflex does not become extensor.

The nerve-fibres of the **sensory neurones** ascend in several different bundles or tracts in the spinal cord and brain-stem to deliver sensory information from all over the body to the cerebral cortex. The fibres carrying crude pain and temperature sense cross almost at once to the opposite side of the spinal cord before turning upwards; those carrying information about the position of the limbs and other parts of the body in space, and those carrying vibration sense and light touch, pass up in the posterior column on the same side and do not cross until they reach the medulla. This anatomical disposition of the tracts explains why a patient with lesion destroying or cutting one half of the spinal cord at a certain level loses the appreciation of pain and temperature on the other side of the body below that level, and vibration sense, position sense and light touch on the same side. Such a patient also of course has an upper motor neurone weakness on the same side below the level of the lesion (see Figure on p. 143).

The Neurological Control of the Bladder and Rectum

The bladder and rectum have a similar nerve-supply and their function may be disturbed by various neurological lesions. In practice disorders of micturition are commoner and more important than disorders of defaecation. The basic nervous mechanism is a sacral reflex arc; when this remains intact and all higher neurological control has been destroyed the bladder is still able to contract and empty itself satisfactorily, but it does this automatically as soon as enough urine has collected to exert a certain critical pressure on the bladder wall. This state of affairs is found in patients who have suffered spinal injury with complete transection of the spinal cord: at

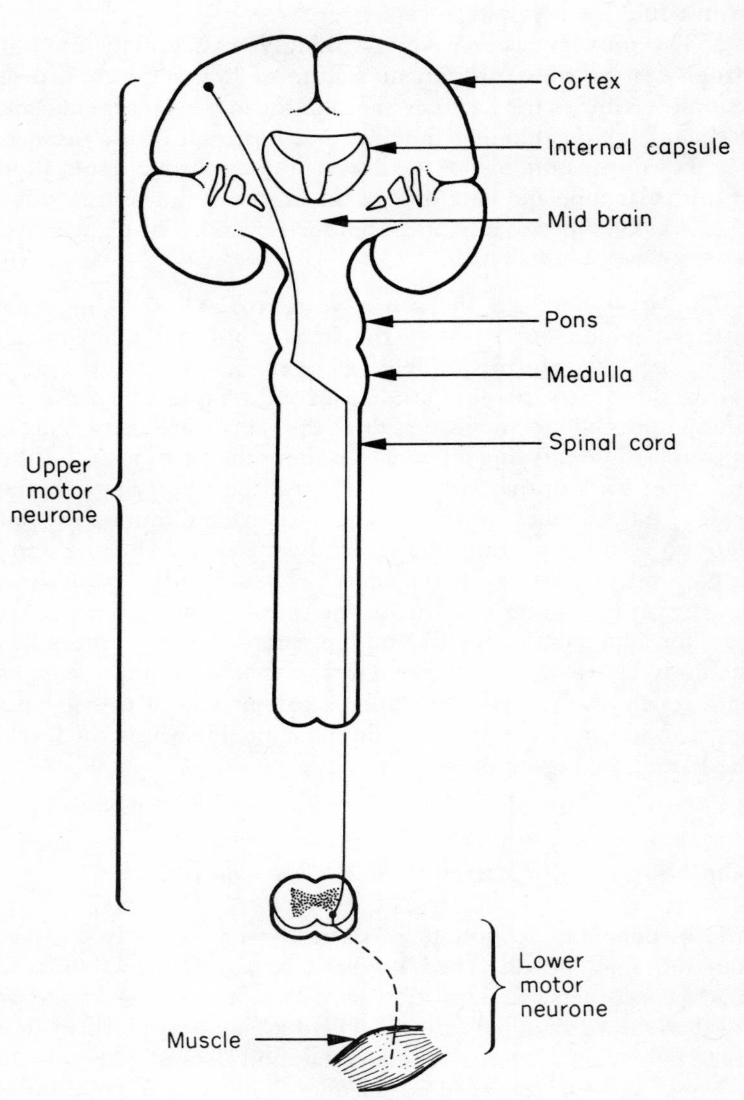
Cortex
Internal capsule
Mid brain
Pons
Medulla
Spinal cord
Upper motor neurone
Lower motor neurone
Muscle

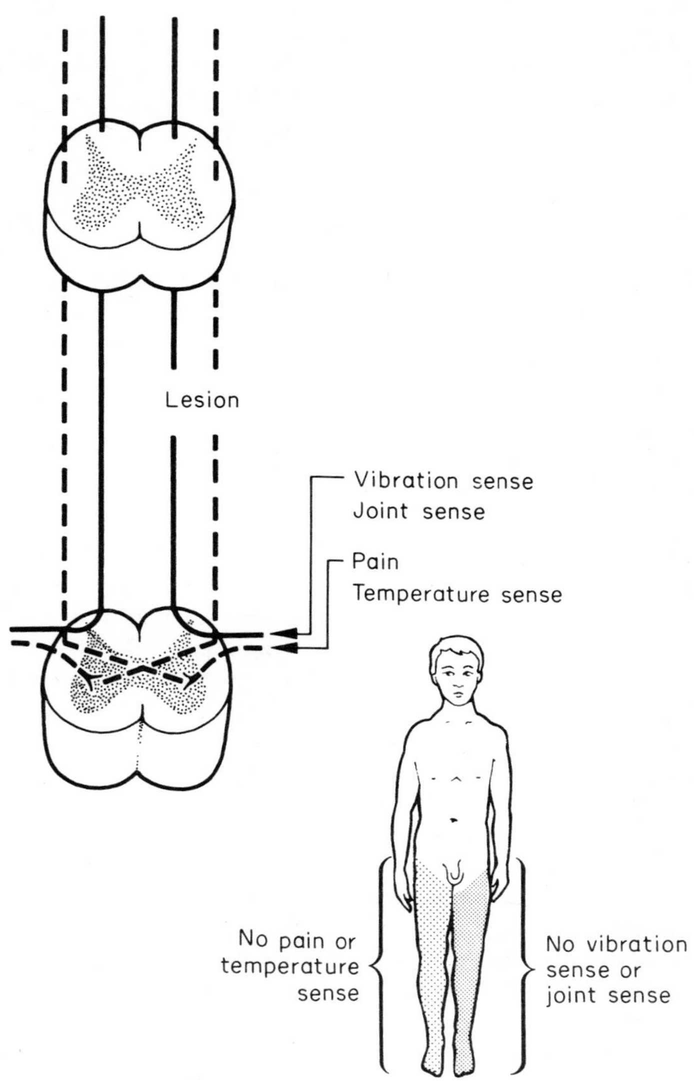

HEMISECTION OF SPINAL CORD

first there is a state of 'spinal shock' for a week or two, during which the bladder does not function at all and the patient has complete retention of urine, but when the stage of shock has passed, the bladder gradually develops the automatic emptying described above. Such patients can often learn in time to avoid wetting themselves by carefully timed use of the bottle, and by attempting to train the bladder to empty itself in response to some stimulus such as scratching the legs.

In a normal person it is the influence of the sympathetic nerve-supply which prevents the automatic evacuation of urine as soon as the bladder is full; while the nerve-fibres carrying voluntary control of micturition enable him to overcome the sympathetic influence and allow the bladder to empty itself. Some diseases of the spinal cord, such as disseminated sclerosis, damage the sympathetic fibres: the patient is therefore unable to hold his water when the bladder is full and suffers from what is called precipitancy of micturition. Other cord diseases affect the voluntary fibres, so that the patient has difficulty in starting the flow of urine or may eventually have complete retention. A disease affecting the first sacral segment of the cord or its nerve-roots, for example tabes dorsalis, interrupts the sacral reflex arc, and in consequence the bladder contracts in a very imperfect and unco-ordinated way and is unable to empty itself completely. As a result there is always some stagnant residual urine in the bladder and urinary infections are very liable to occur.

The Cerebellum exerts a controlling and co-ordinating influence on all the muscular movements of the body, which consequently become wild and uncertain when it is damaged or destroyed. This loss of muscular co-ordination is known as ataxia and it occurs on the same side of the body as the lesion in the cerebellum, though frequently of course the disorder is present on both sides. Ataxia of the ocular muscles causes the oscillating movement of the eyes known as nystagmus; ataxia of the muscles of the larynx and tongue causes a slurred or 'scanning' type of speech; ataxia in the arms is seen as an unsteadiness on movement known as intention tremor; and ataxia of the legs causes a staggering type of gait.

Distinction of Cerebellar Ataxia from Sensory Ataxia

Unsteadiness on movement is sometimes due not to loss of cerebellar control of the muscles but to lack of information about the position of the limbs; this type occurs in diseases like tabes dorsalis and subacute combined degeneration, which destroy the tracts in the spinal cord that normally transmit this information to the brain. Since it is due to loss of the sensory tracts in the posterior column of the spinal cord this type is known as sensory ataxia. Patients deprived in this way of knowledge of the position of their limbs can of course compensate by looking to see where they are; and consequently their ataxia is very much worse when they are in the dark or if they are asked to close their eyes. This is the basis of the Romberg test for distinguishing cerebellar from sensory ataxia. The patient is asked to stand with as good a balance as possible, first with the eyes open and then with the eyes closed; if his ataxia is due to cerebellar disease, the degree of unsteadiness will remain unchanged; but if it is due to lack of sensory impulses from his limbs, removal of the compensatory effect of vision will make him much more unsteady as soon as his eyes are closed.

Diseases of the Central Nervous System

Meningitis

Meningitis means inflammation of the meninges and these, as already pointed out, are the membranes which surround the brain and spinal cord. Usually it is the two inner layers of membrane, the arachnoid and the pia, which become inflamed, and consequently inflammatory changes are found in the CSF, which lies in the space between them.

The type of meningitis varies according to the type of organism causing it. Thus pyogenic organisms (those which cause pus to form) produce an acute pyogenic meningitis in which large numbers of pus cells accumulate in the CSF; the commonest bacteria in this group are the meningococcus, the streptococcus, the staphylococcus and the pneumococcus. Certain viruses also cause an acute meningitis, but they are not pyogenic and the CSF contains not pus but an excess of lymphocytes. More chronic types of meningitis are produced by the tubercle bacillus and the spirochaete of syphilis.

Acute Pyogenic Meningitis

The illness usually starts rather suddenly, often with a shivering attack or actual rigor, soon followed by **fever, severe headache** and **vomiting.** The eyes often become intolerant of light (a symptom known as photophobia). Irritation of the meninges at the base of the brain causes reflex spasm of the muscles at the back of the neck which can be demonstrated by attempting to flex the patient's head forwards. In a normal person the chin can be brought almost in contact with the sternum, but when there is meningeal irritation the muscular spasm prevents any attempt at flexion. This **neck rigidity** is the most important physical sign of meningitis. When the inflammation is very acute the patient may lie with the head drawn well back (in the position of head retraction) and in children the whole body may be arched backwards (in what is called opisthotonos). **Kernig's sign** is also positive in meningitis. To elicit it the leg is first flexed to a right angle at the hip with the knee flexed, and then when an attempt is made to extend the leg at the knee the hamstring muscles go into spasm and the patient complains of pain in the back and neck.

As soon as the diagnosis of acute meningitis has been made lumbar puncture must be done so that the nature of the infecting organism can be determined from examination of the CSF. If the fluid is opaque and turbid the diagnosis of pyogenic meningitis is established, and culture will reveal within a day or so which of the pyogenic bacteria is responsible.

Treatment and Nursing Care Patients with acute meningitis are often drowsy, restless and unco-operative and make great demands therefore on the skill and patience of the nursing staff. In view of the photophobia, the patient may be less restless if kept in a darkened room or in a well-screened-off part of the ward. In addition to the general nursing care the nurse must take particular pains to ensure an adequate fluid intake of some 4 litres daily (for an adult).

Nearly all the pyogenic bacteria are sensitive to sulphonamides and penicillin, and it is usual to start treatment with one or both of these drugs without waiting for the result of the culture. Sulphadiazine is given in an initial dose of 3–4 g, followed by 1 g four-hourly; penicillin is given intramuscularly in doses of about 500 000 units twice daily. This treatment will almost certainly be effective if culture shows that the patient has meningococcal meningitis, which is the commonest variety. If one of the other pyogenic organisms is responsible, it may be advisable to change the treatment to the antibiotic shown to be most suitable by the sensitivity tests done on the organism in the laboratory. Pneumococcal meningitis is usually a complication of a pneumococcal infection elsewhere, particularly pneumonia, and it carries a more serious prognosis than the other types. For this variety it is usually necessary to give penicillin in much larger doses, 4.0 mega-units intravenously every 4 hours for 2 weeks.

Acute Viral (or Lymphocytic) Meningitis

The symptoms and signs are similar to those of pyogenic meningitis, though the patient is usually less gravely ill. The differential diagnosis can only be made with certainty by lumbar puncture, which reveals a clear fluid under slightly increased pressure and containing an excess of lymphocytes. There is no specific treatment and uneventful recovery is the rule.

Tuberculous Meningitis

This is mainly a disease of childhood and adolescence and differs from the acute varieties of meningitis described above in having a slower and more insidious onset. At first the child may simply be vaguely off colour for a week or two, then headache, fever and constipation appear and persist for some days or even longer before neck rigidity and a positive Kernig's sign can be demonstrated. Lumbar puncture reveals a clear fluid under increased pressure, and sometimes a delicate 'cobweb' clot forms in it on standing. Tubercle bacilli can usually be demonstrated in the fluid, which also usually contains an excess of lymphocytes and a diminished content of sugar and chlorides.

Treatment and Nursing Care The choice of drugs used is governed by their ability to pass from the blood into the CSF. The most useful is Isoniazid 10 mg/kg/day given by mouth, combined with pyridoxine 10 mg daily to prevent polyneuritis. In addition streptomycin 1.0 g intramuscularly is usually given daily and rifampicin 12 mg/kg/day orally. In the first month of treatment pyrazinamide 30 mg/kg/day by mouth should be given as well. Streptomycin may damage the vestibular nerve, causing vertigo and ataxia; careful watch must be kept for these symptoms, therefore, and this drug is not usually given for more than 2–3 months, though the isoniazid and rifampicin may be continued for 18 months or two years. Patients should be warned that rifampicin causes reddish discoloration of the urine and reduces the efficacy of the contraceptive pill.

It is extremely important for the patient to be kept at rest, and during the acute stage quiet is essential. He should be nursed in a cubicle or single room, bright light which will aggravate photophobia being avoided.

Being in a wasted condition, the patient is prone to bedsores, and a firm, soft mattress is essential. The position must be changed frequently, and as he usually lies on one side with the hips and knees flexed, particular care should be taken of the skin over these areas. To prevent contractures, regular movements of the joints through their full range is important. During the stage of acute meningeal irritation, movement will be resented; the patient may be very restless, and to prevent injury padded cot sides will be necessary, even for an adult. Sedatives such as chloral or phenobarbitone may be given. Particular care must be given to the mouth, and when the patient is semiconscious or unconscious the eyes should be bathed with normal saline. The danger of inhalation of vomit during this stage must constantly be borne in mind. Constipation may be troublesome and glycerine suppositories or an enema may be used to relieve this condition. Incontinence or retention of urine are not unusual; the latter causes increased restlessness, and catheterisation may be necessary.

Throughout the whole illness an adequate amount of nourishment is essential, and every effort must be made to give a well-balanced diet. The patient may refuse food at first, and feeding by spoon or even by tube may be necessary and requires great patience and perseverance on the part of the nurse; small amounts only will be taken at a time. Vomiting due to cerebral irritation may occur, but food should not be withheld for this reason. A careful record of all nourishment taken must be kept, and after the acute stage the patient should be weighed once a week or oftener.

The acute stage of the illness lasts from six to eight weeks, and gradually the patient begins to feel much better, although he has to remain in bed for many more weeks. Eventually he will be allowed up for short periods, slowly increasing. He must not be allowed to do too much, as there is always a risk of a relapse. The long convalescent stage can be a very difficult one psychologically, particularly if there are disabilities such as deafness or limb paralysis. The patient becomes bored and frustrated, and every effort must be made to keep his mind active without overtiring him. New interests must constantly be introduced.

The almost well child may begin to feel neglected because the nurse is having to spend more time with other seriously ill patients, and so he begins to try to attract attention by being naughty. He may refuse to eat, cry unnecessarily or bite his nails. In the case of a child it is important that the parents visit as often as possible throughout the illness, and during the convalescent stage they should spend more time together to prepare for the patient's return to the family.

Formal education may be commenced long before the child goes home, and the medical social worker will contact the school medical officer if it is necessary for the child to attend a school for physically handicapped children before returning to the strenuous life of an ordinary school. Similar help and advice will be given to the young adult. Careful follow-up with regular examinations of CSF is essential.

Poliomyelitis

Poliomyelitis is a virus infection of the central nervous system which damages the anterior horn cells in the spinal cord and leads therefore to a lower motor neurone type of paralysis. Fortunately the disease is now preventable and has become very rare since immunisation of children became universal; for this purpose 3 drops of oral Sabin vaccine are given on a lump of sugar at 6 months, 7 months, 8 months and 4½ years. The epidemics used to occur in the late summer and autumn. Not all people infected with the virus develop paralysis; some have an illness known as 'abortive' or 'non-paralytic' poliomyelitis, and others remain clinically well but act as healthy carriers and pass the virus on to susceptible contacts. The way in which the disease spreads from one paralysed patient to another is therefore often difficult to trace, since we have no easy way of detecting who the healthy carriers are.The rarity of the disease makes it no longer appropriate to include details of the clinical features and treatment in a book of this scope.

Multiple Sclerosis

This is a disease of unknown cause in which areas of degeneration occur in the central nervous system, particularly in the brain-stem and spinal cord. In most patients the first symptoms appear in early adult life, between the ages of twenty and forty, and women are affected slightly more frequently than men. The disease usually runs a fairly typical course over a number of years; a series of episodes occurs separated by intervals of months or even years, and although the patient makes a partial recovery from each of them, every new episode leaves him with a greater degree of permanent disability, until finally he may become bedridden. Each of these clinical episodes is due to an area of degeneration somewhere in the brain or spinal cord, and the symptoms and signs are therefore very variable, depending on the precise anatomical position of the lesion. The diagnosis often depends therefore not so much on the presence of a typical set of symptoms and signs as on a history of several neurological episodes with intervening remissions of varying length.

However, certain parts of the central nervous system are more commonly affected than others, so that by the time the disease is fairly well established a rather characteristic clinical picture usually emerges. Nearly all patients eventually develop bilateral upper motor neurone lesions in the spinal cord, causing weakness and stiffness in the legs and sometimes in the arms, with very brisk tendon reflexes and extensor plantar responses. Other common lesions are retrobulbar neuritis, causing temporary blindness in one eye, which usually recovers more or less completely in a few days; and a cerebellar lesion, causing nystagmus, slurred or 'scanning' speech and ataxia of the limbs (see p. 144). Disturbance of bladder control, particularly difficulty in holding urine (or precipitancy of micturition), is also common. In the later stages loss of emotional control leads to either laughter or tears on very slight provocation and adds to the distress of both patient and relatives.

Diagnosis The diagnosis of multiple sclerosis depends on a history of a series of neurological episodes and the finding of physical signs of multiple lesions in the brain and spinal cord. It follows that the diagnosis cannot be made with certainty at the time of the initial lesion and it is important that appropriate investigations are done to exclude some other possibly treatable cause for it. There are two tests, however, which may support the diagnosis of MS even at this early stage:

1 The level of the immunoglobulin IgG in the CSF is often raised and the IgG/albumin ratio is higher in the CSF than in the plasma.

2 **Visual and Auditory Evoked Responses**. The response to visual or auditory stimuli is often slower on one side than the other, or than in normal people, revealing the presence of other clinically silent CNS lesions.

Treatment Unfortunately there is no effective specific treatment for multiple sclerosis, but, as already pointed out, the natural tendency is for partial (sometimes almost complete) recovery to occur spontaneously after each clinical episode, so that too gloomy a view must not be taken of the prognosis. This particularly applies to patients in the early stages of the disease, many of whom will in fact enjoy many years (even occasionally a normal lifetime) of quite good health. It must be admitted, however, that in other patients the sum of disabilities piles up quickly over a few years, leading by stages to total incapacity and probably to death before middle age. These unhappy people require the routine nursing care of the helpless patient and, equally important the greatest possible kindness, tact and forbearance on the part of the nurse.

By contacting the medical social worker and making suitable domiciliary arrangements the nurse can help these patients to live comparatively independent and happy lives between the acute stages of the disease. The Multiple Sclerosis Society also provides very valuable help.

Parkinsonism

Parkinsonism is named after Dr. James Parkinson, a general practitioner in London, who described a number of patients with 'the shaking palsy' early last century. It is now recognised that this syndrome may be due to several different diseases which affect the basal ganglia of the brain. The commonest causes are:

1 **Encephalitis.** A certain type of virus infection of the brain may be followed by symptoms and signs of Parkinsonism. This is a disease of early adult life; **postencephalitic Parkinsonism** is almost the only variety which occurs before the age of forty.

2 **Paralysis agitans** is due to degeneration of unknown cause in the cells of the basal ganglia and occurs in late middle age.

3 **Arteriosclerotic Parkinsonism** is due to reduction in the blood supply to the basal ganglia from atheroma of the cerebral arteries. The patients are nearly always over the age of seventy.

4 **A Parkinsonian syndrome** may be a side effect of certain drugs, notably chlorpromazine and haloperidol.

Clinical Features The disease may be limited for a time to one half of the body, but is usually bilateral. The muscles become increasingly **weak** and **rigid,** and in consequence all movements become much slower and very restricted in range. Rigidity of the facial muscles prevents the normal mobility of expression on the face, which becomes set in an unvarying 'Parkinsonian mask'. It is important to remember, however, that although his expressionless face is incapable of revealing his feelings, the patient is often very sensitive and miserable about his progressive disability, and accordingly special care and consideration should be shown to him from this point of view. The muscular rigidity prevents the free swing of the arms in walking, which is often an early sign of the disease, while in the later stages the forward flexion of the whole body and the short, shuffling steps are highly characteristic. Weakness and rigidity of the muscles of the larynx and tongue make the speech slow and rather slurred. The other typical feature is a coarse repetitive **tremor,** which is usually most obvious in the hands. It subsides for a few seconds if the patient makes a voluntary movement such as picking up a pencil, but quickly returns again, and it is made worse by any excitement or emotional stress. It stops during sleep.

As already indicated, the condition is a progressive one, and within a few years most of the patients are more or less completely incapacitated. Sometimes, however, particularly in the younger age groups, the downhill course may be arrested or slowed down, though recovery can never be expected.

Treatment Since the disease is due to destruction of certain neurones in the brain, there can be no cure, and treatment is restricted to the relief of symptoms. The most useful drug is L-dopa, which often greatly facilitates the speed and freedom of muscular movement, but unfortunately its beneficial effect often declines after a few years. Some patients may derive benefit from benzhexol (Artane).

A very small group of patients have severe tremor but very little rigidity, and they may be helped by a neurosurgical operation.

Subacute Combined Degeneration of the Cord

This disease has the same cause as pernicious anaemia (see p. 33), and most of the patients are already suffering from pernicious anaemia before the symptoms and signs appear. The primary lesion is atrophy of the stomach, which is consequently unable to absorb enough vitamin B12 for the adequate nourishment of the blood and spinal cord. The atrophic stomach also fails to secrete acid into the gastric juice; and demonstration by fractional test meal that the patient has no acid in his stomach, even after having been given histamine 0.5 mg subcutaneously, is an essential part of the investigation of the disease. If he has acid in his stomach he cannot have either PA or subacute combined degeneration.

The parts of the nervous system which degenerate when starved of vitamin B12 are the posterior and lateral columns of the spinal cord (hence the term 'combined degeneration') and certain peripheral nerves. Degeneration of the latter usually gives rise to the earliest symptoms of numbness and tingling or pins and needles (so-called paraesthesiae) in the feet and hands. Later the posterior column degeneration leads to loss of joint sense and vibration sense and to unsteadiness of the legs, which is worse when the eyes are closed (see 'sensory ataxia', p. 144); and the lateral column lesion damages the upper motor neurone causing weakness of the limbs and extensor plantar responses.

Treatment The patient must be given injections of vitamin B12 or liver extract regularly for the rest of his life, the dosage and frequency of injections being decided on the results of regular blood counts. If enough B12 is not given to keep the blood normal there is grave danger that the spinal cord will suffer further damage; and whereas the anaemia and the peripheral nerve lesion may recover completely under treatment, the spinal cord degeneration is permanent.

Cerebral Tumours

Cerebral tumours may be primary, if they arise from some intracranial structure, or secondary, if they arise from malignant cells carried in the bloodstream to the brain from elsewhere in the body. Common examples of primary tumours are meningiomas, which arise from the meninges and, being therefore on the surface of the brain, are relatively easy to remove; neurofibromas, which grow on the cranial nerves and are particularly common on the eighth cranial nerve; and gliomas, which are rather malignant tumours, arising from the interstitial tissue of the brain substance and which in consequence are usually inoperable. Secondary carcinoma in the brain is nearly always due to spread from a primary carcinoma of the bronchus.

Clinical Features The symptoms and signs arise in two ways:

1 Owing to the fact that the tumour occupies space inside the skull, all the normal structures are somewhat compressed and there

is a **raised intracranial pressure.** This causes **headache,** which is often very severe and is made worse by lying down or coughing or straining in any way; **vomiting,** particularly when the patient gets up in the morning; and **papilloedema,** or swelling of the optic nerve seen through an ophthalmoscope. This combination of headache, vomiting and papilloedema is a very important indication of raised intracranial pressure, and should always lead to further investigation of the cause. Symptoms which may also occur in these patients are attacks of vertigo (dizziness) or epileptic fits.

2 Other symptoms and signs may be due to direct pressure by the tumour on some part of the brain. An eighth nerve tumour, for example, causes deafness on that side as well as other signs of local pressure, and tumours of the pituitary compress the visual nerve-fibres (in the optic chiasma) and cause blindness in part of the visual field.

Investigations Lumbar puncture may reveal that the CSF pressure is raised (the normal range of pressure is about 50–160 mm), and analysis of the fluid usually shows an increased protein content (normal range about 30–50 mg per 100 ml). It is very important to remember, however, that lumbar puncture may be dangerous in patients with raised intracranial pressure, as the release of fluid from the lumbar subarachnoid space may cause the brain-stem to be pushed down into the foramen magnum, with grave risk of death from compression of the vital centres in the medulla. **X-ray of the skull** may show certain changes resulting from the raised intracranial pressure. **Cerebral arteriogram** is an X-ray taken after injecting a dye into the carotid or vertebral arteries to make the vessels of the brain visible. Certain brain tumours produce evidence of their presence by distorting the normal pattern of blood vessels in that region. X-rays may be taken after filling the ventricles (or cavities in the brain) with air to make them visible. The air may be introduced directly through a needle passed through a burr-hole made in the skull and then through the brain itself into the lateral ventricle; this procedure is called **ventriculography.** Alternatively the air may be introduced into the lumbar subarachnoid space through an ordinary lumbar puncture needle and then made to rise into the ventricles of the brain by standing the patient up; this is called **air encephalography.** By either technique it may be shown that the tumour has caused distortion or displacement of the ventricles of the brain, an observation which helps to localise it. In some cases the electro-encephalogram (EEG) shows abnormal waves from the area of the skull overlying the tumour. Two newer non-invasive techniques have greatly reduced the indications for arteriography and air studies, which are not without danger. These are (1) **Brain Scan.** An injected isotope, technetium 99^m, is taken up by abnormal structures such as tumours and reveals them on X-ray. (2) **Computerised Tomography** (by the EMI Scanner) is a very sophisticated type of radiography which reveals the intracranial structures in remarkable detail.

Treatment The only hope of cure lies in surgical removal of the tumour. If this cannot be done the patient is likely to suffer progressively severe headaches, vomiting, perhaps failure of vision and eventually paralysis, and increasing doses of morphine or allied drugs are necessary when the symptoms become severe.

Neurosyphilis

Syphilis attacks the nervous system in the tertiary stage many years after the infection has been acquired, so that apart from rare cases in childhood due to congenital infection, the patients are mostly middle-aged. It is several times commoner in men than in women. There are three main varieties: meningovascular syphilis, tabes dorsalis and GPI (general paralysis of the insane).

Meningovascular syphilis is so called because of the chronic inflammatory changes which occur in the meninges and in the arteries which supply the brain and spinal cord with blood. The meninges become thickened and the affected arteries become very much narrowed (by a process known as 'endarteritis obliterans') and in consequence certain neurones in the brain and spinal cord die from lack of oxygen. The clinical symptoms and signs are very variable, therefore, and depend on which particular arteries are diseased, so that meningovascular syphilis can mimic almost any other disease of the central nervous system. For this reason it is usual to do a serological test for syphilis in the course of the investigation of all neurological patients.

Tabes Dorsalis means literally 'dorsal wasting', and refers to the atrophy that occurs in the nerve-fibres in the posterior columns of the spinal cord, which normally carry position sense, vibration sense and light touch. The loss of position sense causes the characteristic ataxia of tabes, which is worse in the dark or when the eyes are closed (see p. 144). Since the patient also cannot feel the normal pressure of the ground on the soles of his feet, he brings them down with excessive force, hence the typical 'stamping' gait. Irritation of the posterior nerve-roots entering the spinal cord causes 'lightning pains', which shoot down the legs like recurring flashes of lightning and then often disappear for a week or two. They sometimes seem to come back with a change in the weather, and many patients therefore erroneously attribute them to 'rheumatism'. Destruction of the first sacral nerve-root interrupts the reflex arc which controls micturition and results in inability to empty the bladder properly (see p. 144); while destruction of the roots at S1 and 2 and L2, 3 and 4 abolish the ankle-jerk and the knee-jerk respectively. Another common finding in tabetics is Argyll-Robertson pupils, which are small, unequal, irregular and fail to contract on exposure to light, though they still react in accommodation. This abnormality of the pupils, together with slight lowering of the upper lids (ptosis) and wrinkling of the forehead, sometimes produces a characteristic tabetic facial appearance (or facies).

Because of the sensory loss, so-called trophic lesions may occur in the limbs from a succession of minor injuries which the patient cannot feel and against which no protective reflexes operate. The perforating ulcer starts as an abrasion on the sole of the foot; as it is painless the patient continues to walk on it, and it may develop into a deep ulcer which finally perforates through to the dorsum of the foot. The Charcot joint is a severe but painless osteo-arthritis which causes great destruction of the joint surfaces and may eventually lead to dislocation. The knee is the joint most commonly affected.

Other important complications are urinary infection due to imperfect emptying of the bladder and the gastric crisis, which is an attack of severe abdominal pain and vomiting due to irritation of nerve-roots in the thoracic region of the cord.

About 70–80 per cent of tabetics have a positive test for syphilis in the blood or CSF, and the latter nearly always shows a positive Lange test.

Treatment The ataxia of tabes is always very much worse after a period of confinement to bed, and these patients must therefore be kept on their feet unless there is some imperative reason for complete rest. If it is thought that the syphilis is still active an intensive course of penicillin should be given. The urine must be examined frequently for pus cells, since loss of bladder sensation prevents the usual frequency and pain of urinary infection, which can therefore easily be overlooked. If there is evidence of infection the urine should be cultured and a course of treatment given with an antibiotic appropriate to the organism isolated. The ataxia can often be improved to a remarkable extent by a course of re-educative exercises given under the guidance of a physiotherapist.

GPI is the rarest type of neurosyphilis and results from destruction of nerve-cells in the cerebral cortex by spirochaetes which have invaded the brain. The first symptoms are mental; a progressive deterioration in intellect occurs and the patient starts making mistakes in his work. He remains unaware of his failing mental powers, however, and it is usually a relative or business colleague who first seeks medical advice on his behalf. Indeed, the patient himself may have delusions of grandeur and imagine himself to be a person of great wealth, power and importance. In time physical symptoms and signs also appear, many of them being due to destruction of upper motor neurone cells in both cerebral hemispheres. The patient therefore has a progressive spastic weakness of the limbs, with exaggeration of the tendon reflexes and extensor plantar responses. He also develops a coarse tremor of the lips and hands, slurring of speech and Argyll-Robertson pupils. Epileptiform fits are common. Tests for syphilis are always positive in the blood and CSF, and the Lange test is also positive in the CSF.

Treatment GPI is a progressive disease, and in the absence of treatment leads to complete paralysis, dementia and finally death within a year or two. On the other hand, if treatment is given early enough the patient may be sufficiently restored both mentally and physically to be able to resume his previous occupation. Early diagnosis and treatment are therefore of the greatest importance. At the present time the latter consists simply of an intensive course of penicillin, which it may be necessary to repeat once or twice if subsequent examination of the patient and his CSF reveals signs that the disease may still be active.

Tetanus

The tetanus bacilli, *Clostridium tetani*, is found in horse manure, cultivated soil and road dust, and human infection is acquired from contamination of wounds. Since the organism is anaerobic (grows best in the absence of oxygen), deep puncture wounds are more likely to be complicated by tetanus than superficial surface abrasions. The symptoms and signs of the disease appear when the powerful toxin produced by the organisms in the wound have travelled up the peripheral nerves and reach the central nervous system. The interval between the occurrence of the wound and the appearance of the tetanic symptoms varies from two or three days to two or three weeks; a short interval indicates a virulent infection and therefore a poor prognosis.

Symptoms Pain and stiffness of the muscles of the jaw and neck are usually the first indication of the disease, trismus (inability to open the mouth) being a very characteristic early symptom. Fixed contraction of the facial muscles may draw the angles of the mouth apart in the semblance of a smile, known as the 'risus sardonicus'. Within a day or two the muscles of the trunk and limbs are also in a state of painful spasm, and the fact that the mind remains quite clear and alert makes the condition a particularly distressing one. At this stage any external stimulus may send the whole body into a powerful reflex spasm which arches it backwards into a state of opisthotonos and causes a great increase in pain. Tetanus has a high mortality rate, death being due mainly to respiratory paralysis, exhaustion or pneumonia.

Treatment Specially staffed and equipped tetanus units have been established in Britain and strenuous efforts should be made to have the patient transferred without delay to the nearest of these. He should be nursed in a quiet room with shaded light. Human antitetanus immunoglobulin (Humotet, Wellcome) is the antitoxin of choice since it avoids the serious allergic reactions which may follow horse serum antitoxin; the dose is 30–300 IU/kg body weight, given intramuscularly. The antitoxin neutralises any new toxin formed at the site of infection, but is unfortunately unable to affect toxin which has already reached the central nervous system. It is necessary also to give large doses of sedatives to control the muscular spasms; chlorpromazine 50–100 mg intravenously followed by 50–100 mg intramuscularly every 4–6 hours may be given for this purpose.

If muscular spasms continue, a muscle relaxant such as curare with an anaesthetic such as thiopentone may be needed to relieve them; such patients must be under continuous observation by a doctor, since the patient may require mechanical respiration to maintain life.

The wound should not be excised until several hours after the intravenous injection of antitoxin, as the disturbance of the wound may cause fresh toxin to escape into the bloodstream.

Nursing Care When nursing such a patient every effort must be made to eliminate anything which will provoke a muscular spasm. The patient is nursed in a darkened room as far away from noise as possible. Absolute quiet should be observed, since even the opening and closing of a door will worry the patient and only essential medical and nursing personnel should be admitted. Mental alertness is acute and the patient is anxious and frightened. He will naturally resent and fear movement and everything must be done to allay fear and gain his confidence. Speech may also be affected and the nurse must try to anticipate his needs. Nursing care is timed to be carried out to coincide with the maximum effect of the sedatives. The patient's position will be changed and pressure areas treated. Washing is reduced to the minimum. Three people should lift the patient when changing the position and any necessary bedmaking will be done at that time. The nurse must always make sure her hands are warm when handling the patient.

As already said, severe spasms may be controlled by use of muscle relaxants and thiopentone and then the nursing care will be as for any unconscious patient.

Because of trismus and fear, feeding is a problem from the onset. At first oral feeding may be possible and fluids with glucose added should be given freely. When this method becomes impossible other means will have to be adopted. While the patient is under the influence of drugs, passing a nasal tube into the oesophagus and leaving it in situ will be the most satisfactory method; needless to say, the greatest care must be taken to ensure that it does not pass by mistake into the larynx and trachea.

Care of the mouth is important; salivation may be excessive and suction will have to be used when swallowing is difficult and while the patient is unconscious. Atropine may be given to dry up the secretions.

The patient sweats profusely during a spasm and must be carefully sponged and dried whenever necessary. The temperature will be taken per rectum twice daily, but more frequent observations of the pulse have to be made, as the heart rate is usually very fast.

In patients who recover, the muscle spasms gradually diminish and general improvement follows. Stiffness may remain for some weeks and physiotherapy will be of value during convalescence.

Prevention 1 **Active Immunisation** This is achieved by three intramuscular injections of tetanus toxoid 1 ml at intervals of 3 weeks.

2 **Passive Immunisation** All non-immunised patients with tetanus-prone wounds should be given antitoxin. Human anti-tetanus immunoglobulin (Humotet, Wellcome) should be used,

since it provides better protection and has none of the disadvantages of horse serum antitoxin; the dose is 250–500 IU intramuscularly. At the same time the first immunising dose of adsorbed toxoid should be given.

Vascular Disorders of the Brain

Atheroma is a common disease of the cerebral arteries in middle-aged and elderly people, particularly in those who have a raised blood pressure. It causes a progressive narrowing of the arteries, and in consequence of the reduction in blood supply the functions of the brain show a steady decline. These patients therefore become mentally sluggish, their memory becomes poor, particularly for recent events, they often become rather irritable and 'difficult', and in the later stages they gradually lose control of the bladder and rectum. This 'second childhood' may last for several years and is a period of sadness and distress for the relatives and friends. The patient is likely to retain his faculties best in the familiar surroundings of his own home and often becomes much more confused and helpless if he has to be admitted to hospital, so that he should not be moved until this is absolutely necessary. Similarly, the downhill progress is much more rapid in those who do not keep themselves mentally and physically active, so that every effort should be made to encourage any occupation within the patient's powers to postpone as long as possible the final stage of confinement to bed. It must be recognised, however, that such a patient is often a considerable burden on his family, and if there is no one able (or willing) to look after him there may be no alternative to removing him to an institution.

Apoplectic Strokes are sudden catastrophes due to cerebral haemorrhage, cerebral thrombosis or cerebral embolism. The first two, haemorrhage and thrombosis, are usually complications of cerebral atheroma and occur therefore in elderly people; cerebral embolism is plugging of a patent and often healthy cerebral artery by a piece of blood-clot or vegetation detached from the heart, either from the left atrium in patients with mitral stenosis and atrial fibrillation or from a 'mural thrombus' in the left ventricle in patients who have had a recent myocardial infarct.

All three produce a similar type of stroke, though the clinical features vary somewhat from case to case according to the particular cerebral artery affected. Haemorrhage occurs mainly in people with high blood pressure and atheroma, and it often occurs at the height of some muscular effort, such as straining at stool, which raises the blood pressure still higher. The patient rapidly loses consciousness, the depth of coma becomes progressively deeper over the next day or two, and death is the usual outcome. Cerebral thrombosis is less often associated with hypertension, the onset is often rather gradual while the patient is at rest, consciousness is not necessarily lost, and most patients make at least a partial recovery over a period of some weeks. Cerebral embolism has an extremely abrupt onset in a patient with heart disease, either mitral stenosis with auricular fibrillation, bacterial endocarditis or myocardial infarction with a mural thrombus (see p. 22); consciousness is usually lost; but some degree of eventual recovery is the rule.

A patient who has had a severe stroke with coma passes first into a state of cerebral shock in which the limbs are flaccid and the head and eyes are often deviated to one side. The breathing is often noisy (stertorous) and the paralysed cheek on the side opposite to the lesion may be seen to blow in and out with the movements of respiration. In patients destined to recover, consciousness gradually returns over a day or two and it now becomes apparent that there is weakness (paresis) or complete paralysis in the arm and leg (i.e. a hemiplegia) on the opposite side to the lesion. Right-handed patients with a right-sided paralysis, and left-handed patients with a left-sided paralysis usually also show loss of speech (aphasia); this is because the motor centre for speech lies in the left cerebral hemisphere in right-handed people and in the right cerebral hemisphere in left-handed people. Within about a week, when the signs of cerebral shock have completely passed off, the signs of an upper motor neurone lesion can be found on the side of the hemiplegia; the weak arm and leg become stiff and spastic, the tendon reflexes on that side are exaggerated and the plantar response is extensor. From now on there is a gradual recovery both in the power of speech and in the limbs, and how complete this will be depends on the size of the vascular lesion in the brain. Power returns to the leg before the arm, and fine movements of the fingers are usually the last to recover; many patients are left with a more or less severe permanent spastic weakness.

Nursing Care of Hemiplegia The nursing of such a patient calls for the greatest degree of skill and ingenuity. The paralysed patient is going to be helpless and largely dependent on others for a long time, and the nurse will have to care not only for the physical needs but help in the social and psychological rehabilitation.

In the early stages the patient, if unconscious, is nursed on the unaffected side to prevent the tongue from falling back and causing obstruction and to allow saliva to trickle out of the mouth. A pillow is placed at the back to give support, and the arm and leg should also be adequately supported. Change of position is essential, as these patients are particularly prone to bedsores and hypostatic pneumonia. If available, alternating pressure beds are advantageous, but do not minimise the need for basic nursing care of pressure areas.

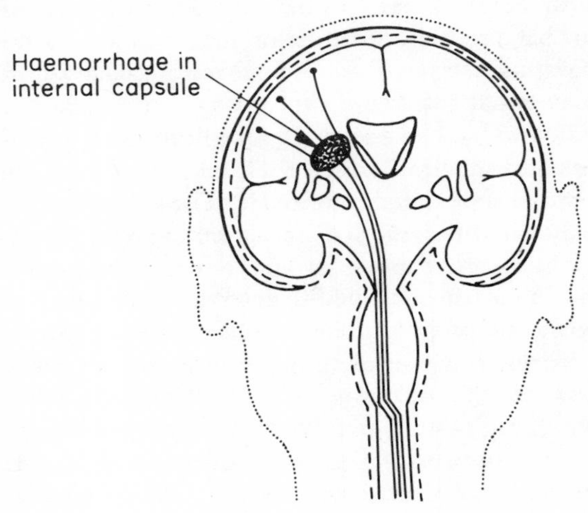

Haemorrhage into the internal capsule (or thrombosis or embolism of the artery supplying it) damages the upper motor neurones which carry the impulses for voluntary movement to the opposite half of the body and so causes hemiplegia.

If the patient is unconscious for more than a few hours, fluid should be given per rectum. Later it will be necessary to give nourishing fluids by nasal tube until the patient is able to swallow.

Incontinence or retention of urine may occur. The latter is dealt with by insertion of a self-retaining catheter. Retention with overflow must not be confused with true incontinence, and a restless, unconscious patient should be catheterised to ascertain that the bladder is being emptied. The strictest aseptic technique is necessary, as cystitis is likely to occur. Constipation of two days' standing should be relieved by giving an enema.

Nursing care is aimed at the prevention of contractures and at restoration of function. The patient is placed in the dorsal position with the head and shoulders slightly raised, but flexion of the head must be avoided. Gradually the patient is brought into a semi-upright position, taking great care to give support to the small of the back, the head and shoulders.

When dealing with paralysed limbs, it should be remembered that they must be supported in the position of maximum function to counteract the deformities caused by spasticity. As already mentioned, the period of flaccidity is followed by spasticity. Fatigue and overstretching of weak muscles must be avoided.

During the flaccid stage the paralysed arm should be abducted. A pillow placed lengthways under it, extending well up into the axilla and supporting the shoulder joint, will prevent contraction of axillary muscles. A roll of cotton wool or a bandage is placed in the palm of the hand and the fingers are arranged in a grasping position. The wrist is placed in the position of slight dorsiflexion by use of a small pillow or a light plaster cock-up splint. To prevent involuntary adduction a firm pillow can be placed between the patient's chest and arm. As an alternative method the arm can be suspended in a canvas sling in a position of abduction.

Care of the Paralysed Leg External rotation of the leg must be prevented by supporting the hip. A firm pad should be placed against the outer aspect of the thigh, extending from above the hip to below the knee. To prevent strain on the abdominal muscles and tension on the calf muscles a pillow or sorbo pad is placed under the knee. The foot is held in a position of dorsiflexion by use of a good foot support. A sorbo pad is placed under the lower part of the leg to prevent pressure on the heel. If a foot-board is used it will also take the weight of the bedclothes, and so prevent restriction of toe movement; otherwise a bed-cradle will be necessary.

It will be necessary to change the patient's position on to the unaffected side to relieve pressure and prevent pulmonary congestion. When moving the limbs the nurse must support them gently under the joints.

To prevent adhesions forming in and around the joints and to prevent circulatory stagnation, passive movements should be commenced a few days after the onset, paralysed limbs being put through the full range of movement two or three times a day (see Figure on pp. 165–6). Breathing exercises must also be given at every opportunity.

Fluids and Diet When one side of the patient's face is paralysed and swallowing is difficult, feeding of the patient is not an easy matter. Polythene tubing or a straw may facilitate taking of fluids. The patient's head should be turned to the unaffected side to prevent

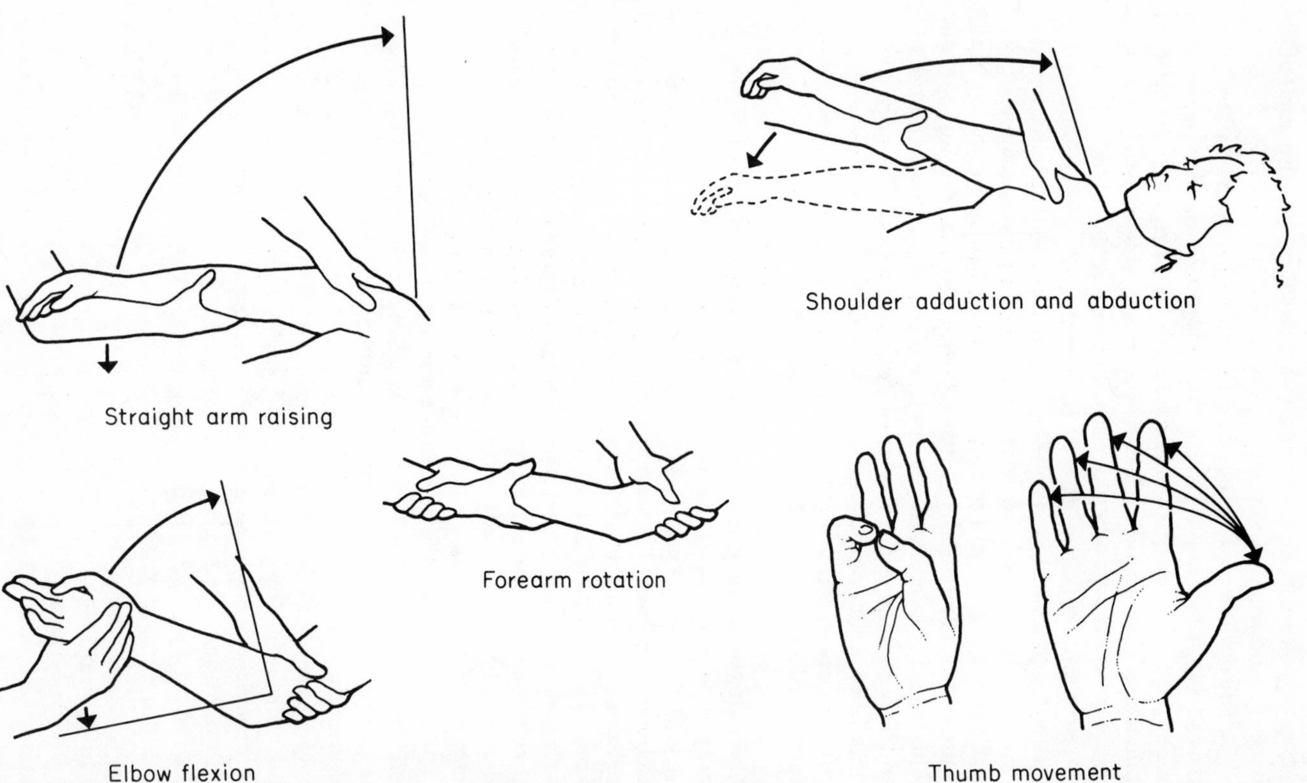

Shoulder adduction and abduction

Straight arm raising

Elbow flexion

Forearm rotation

Thumb movement

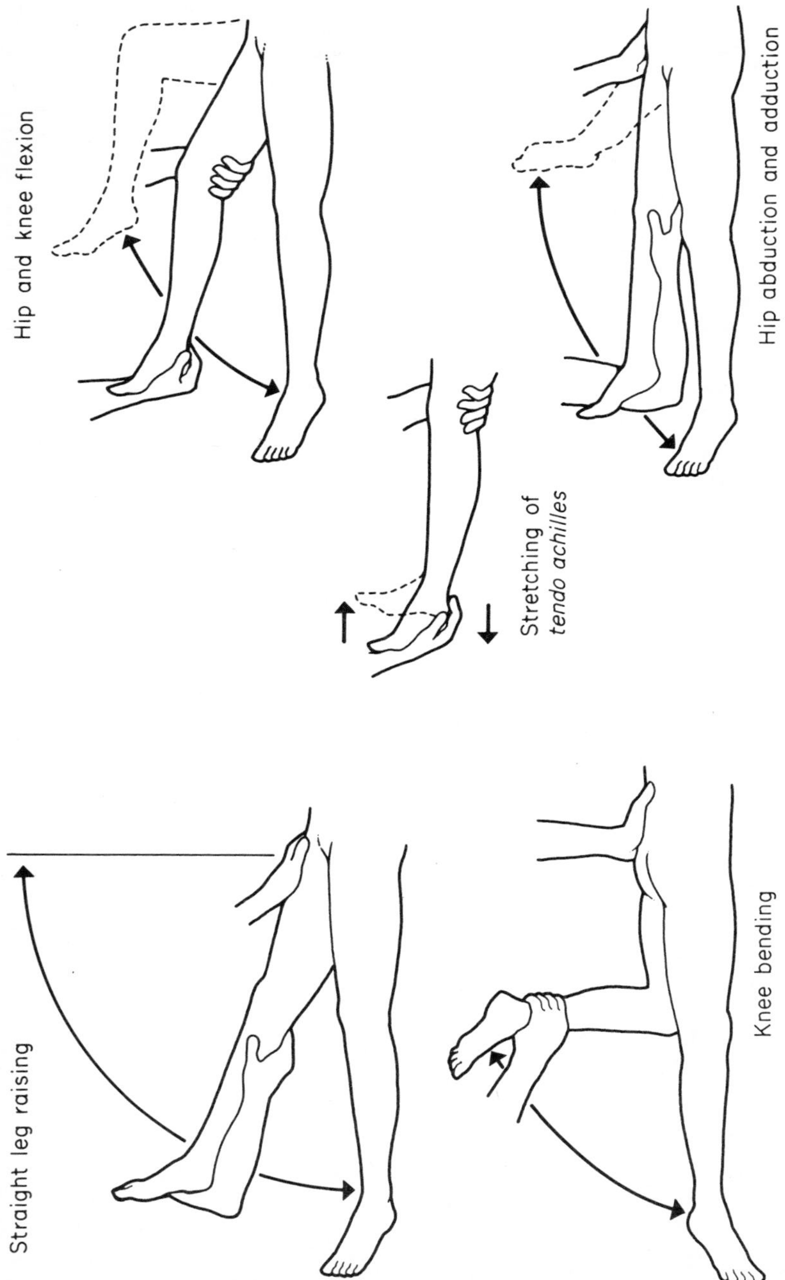
Hip and knee flexion
Hip abduction and adduction
Stretching of *tendo achilles*
Straight leg raising
Knee bending

any particles of food lodging in the paralysed part of the mouth; a dental syringe is useful to dislodge particles of food. The patient's morale will be helped by encouraging him to feed himself as soon as possible, and padding the handle of his spoon may facilitate this.

Aphasia Disturbance of speech is one of the most distressing features, and unfortunately the patient may not be able to write down his needs. The importance of the nurse anticipating his wants is obvious. The patient's emotional state may also be affected, and untiring patience and understanding are necessary on the part of the nursing staff. Speech therapy is often necessary, as he may have to be taught to speak as if he were a child.

Voluntary Movement As soon as there is any sign of voluntary movement every encouragement must be given, to the extent of putting the unaffected arm in a sling, thus forcing him to use the affected one. Occupational and recreational therapy will also be of value. The patient is got out of bed as soon as possible and encouraged to walk; assistance will be needed at first, but gradually the use of a stick will be sufficient. He will often be depressed because progress is slow, and the nurse must do all she can to keep him cheerful. Such a patient will have a dread of being dependent on relatives, and every effort must be made to help him to become independent, and his family should be taught how they can help by continual encouragement and understanding. Innumerable gadgets are available which will help him to overcome his disability.

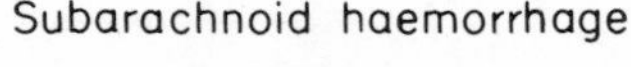

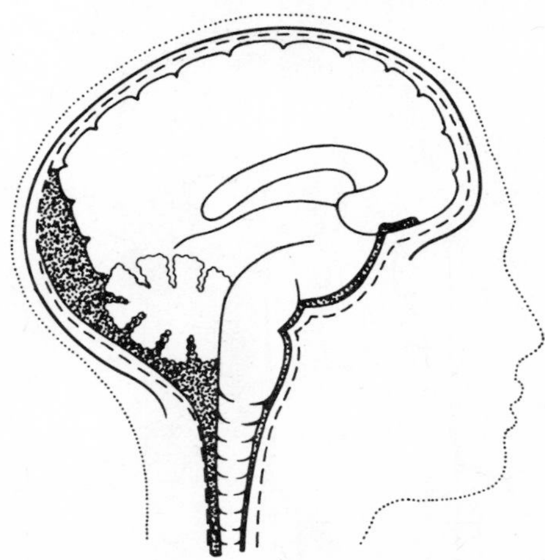

Rupture of a Congenital Aneurysm on an artery at the base of the brain causes **subarachnoid haemorrhage,** which is an uncommon type of stroke occurring in young adults. There is sudden onset of severe pain at the back of the head, followed by drowsiness or coma, and on examination signs of meningeal irritation (neck stiffness and a positive Kernig's sign) are found. The condition is distinguished from acute meningitis by the abrupt onset and the absence of fever and the presence of blood in the CSF establishes the diagnosis. Gradual recovery occurs in about two-thirds of the patients, but subsequent bleeding is always a danger and some neurosurgeons advocate operation to try to prevent this.

Chronic Subdural Haematoma is a rare type of intracranial haemorrhage due to tearing of the small veins which run between the arachnoid and the dura mater, and it often follows quite a trivial head injury which is not regarded by the patient as of any particular importance at the time. The slow collection of blood between the dura and the arachnoid causes increasing pressure on the underlying cerebral hemisphere on the affected side, and leads after a week or two to headache and slight mental confusion. The headache may eventually be severe and associated with vomiting; the patient gradually loses interest in his surroundings and becomes increasingly drowsy, and at this stage striking fluctuations in the degree of impairment of consciousness occur from day to day. Death may follow unless the blood is evacuated by surgical exploration, in which case complete recovery is the rule.

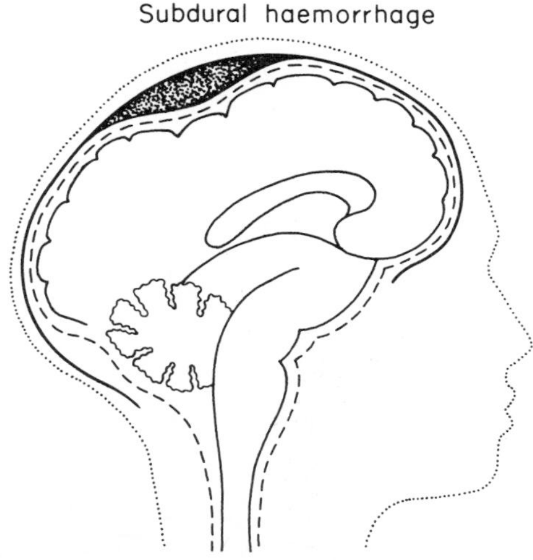

Epilepsy

Epilepsy is a condition in which from time to time bursts of abnormal impulses are discharged from part of the brain and cause fits of various kinds. From a clinical point of view epilepsy is divided into symptomatic and idiopathic varieties.

Symptomatic Epilepsy is so called because the periodic bursts of impulses are due to irritation of the brain by some other disease, and the fits are therefore simply a symptom of that disease. There are many diseases which may affect the brain in this way; they include not only lesions within the skull, such as cerebral tumour, GPI, cerebral vascular lesions and the effects of head injury, which irritate the cortex directly, but also more general diseases such as uraemia from renal failure, in which the abnormal stimulus to the brain is supplied by accumulated poisons in the blood.

Idiopathic Epilepsy. The word 'idiopathic' applied to a disease means that its cause is not known. In idiopathic epilepsy the brain is anatomically normal, though an abnormality in the electric waves discharged by it can be demonstrated on the electro-encephalogram (EEG). These patients probably inherit their tendency to epilepsy, and there is often a history of fits in other members of the family.

Epileptic Fits may take many forms, but the most important varieties are the major fit ('grand mal'), the minor fit ('petit mal') and the Jacksonian fit.

The Major Fit is sometimes preceded by a momentary sensation (or aura) which the patient comes to recognise as a warning that he is about to have an attack, but usually there is no warning at all. The fit starts with what is called the 'tonic stage': there is sudden loss of consciousness and the patient falls to the ground with all his muscles in a state of increased tone. Since the muscular spasm holds the whole body rigid, the patient falls heavily, and may split his scalp or injure himself in some other way; and if he is in a position of special danger he may kill himself or others. For this reason known epileptics should not be allowed to work with dangerous machinery or at a height and it is illegal for them to hold a driving licence. Since the movements of respiration stop during the tonic stage, the patient becomes cyanosed, and this helps to distinguish the epileptic seizure from a simple faint (or syncopal attack), in which the patient becomes very pale. The tonic stage lasts only a matter of seconds, not more than half a minute, and is followed by the 'clonic stage', in which the muscles which have been in a state of rigid spasm go through a series of convulsive movements. This stage also lasts up to half a minute. During it evacuation of the bladder and less often the rectum may occur, and saliva which has collected in the mouth may be lathered up into a froth on the lips by the movements of the jaw and tongue. When the convulsions stop, the patient remains in coma with the muscles relaxed; if he is examined at this stage the corneal and tendon reflexes are found to be absent and the plantar responses extensor. Most patients recover consciousness in a few minutes, though occasionally the coma may last for several hours. Status epilepticus is the condition in which a patient has a series of convulsions without intervening recovery of consciousness; it is always serious and may prove fatal if intensive treatment is not given. On coming round the patient nearly always complains of severe headache, and very occasionally he spends the next few hours in a curious state rather like sleep-walking, known as 'post-epileptic automatism', in which he may perform embarrassing or illegal acts without knowing what he is doing.

Petit Mal is simply a sudden clouding of consciousness lasting a few seconds. It shows itself as a sudden stop in conversation or whatever else the patient is doing at the time, and usually he does not fall down, but quickly comes to and resumes where he left off.

The Jacksonian Fit consists of a convulsion starting in one part of the body, such as the thumb, angle of mouth or foot, without loss of consciousness. Sometimes the attack remains localised, but more often the movements spread up the limb in an orderly fashion and eventually become generalised, and when they cross to involve the other side of the body the patient passes into coma. Such an attack suggests that the epileptic focus in the brain lies in the part of the cortex which controls movement in the segment of the limb first involved by the fit.

Treatment If the patient has symptomatic epilepsy, then obviously treatment must be given for the disease which is causing the fits. A patient in status epilepticus must of course receive the care necessary for any unconscious patient, and in addition he must be given large doses of sedatives to bring the convulsions under control. The drug of choice is diazepam (Valium) 10 mg by slow IV injection; this may be repeated as necessary until control is achieved.

Prevention of fits can be achieved in the vast majority of epileptics by giving an anticonvulsant drug in sufficient dosage to maintain its level in the blood in the upper part of the therapeutic range. It is much better to give a single drug in adequate dosage than to prescribe combinations of drugs. The drug of first choice is Phenytoin; it is usual to start with 200 mg, given as a single daily dose or as 100 mg b.d., and to increase the dose slowly until the blood level lies towards the upper part of the therapeutic range of 3–16 mg/l. Other drugs in common use are Carbamazepine (starting dose 200 mg per day; therapeutic range in blood 4–14 mg/l); Valproate (starting dose 600 mg per day; therapeutic range in blood 40–80 mg/l) and Primidone (starting dose 500 mg per day; therapeutic range in blood: up to 14 mg/l). Phenobarbitone is now seldom given as an anticonvulsant because it tends to cause behavioural disturbance in children and sedation and depression in adults. In a small proportion of severe epileptics the fits cannot be well enough controlled to enable them to lead normal lives, and they require special management in epileptic colonies.

Epilepsy and Driving By definition epilepsy is a liability to recurrent fits; a single epileptic seizure therefore does not warrant the diagnosis epilepsy. When this diagnosis is made UK law does not permit the patient to hold a driving licence until he has been free from attacks for three years.

Hysteria

Hysteria is a very common psychological illness which occurs in people who are physically healthy but also produces symptoms in patients suffering from organic disease. The tendency to hysteria is part of the patient's personality, or, to put it another way, hysterics are born and not made. People with this tendency are naïve and immature, emotionally shallow and extremely suggestible, and they lack the ability to face up to life's difficulties and make decisions which are painful, embarrassing or distasteful. When placed in a dilemma from which he can see no satisfactory escape, or in a situation where what he wants to do conflicts with what he feels he ought to do, the hysteric is unable to decide on a plan of action and face whatever consequences there may be; instead he develops a hysterical illness which serves the purpose of withdrawing him from the situation which he finds intolerable. Every hysterical symptom, therefore, is serving some purpose for the patient, but it is a subconscious purpose. Deliberate pretence of illness to escape some tiresome duty is malingering; hysterical illness has a similar effect, but the psychological processes leading to it take place below the level of consciousness and the patient is unaware of them.

Hysterical symptoms are of many different types, but nearly all of them seem to be produced by a cutting off from consciousness of some part of the patient's experience. When this process operates at the psychological level the patient passes into what is called a 'hysterical fugue': that is, he suffers complete loss of memory, does not know his name or address and is quite cut off from his previous life. More commonly the cutting-off process operates at the physical level and the patient suffers complete loss of some function of his body. Common examples are hysterical blindness, hysterical deafness, hysterical aphonia (loss of voice) and hysterical paralysis or anaesthesia (loss of feeling) in one or more limbs. It should be stressed that the patient does not simply pretend that he cannot see, hear, speak, feel or move his limb; these functions are genuinely lost to him for the time being; for example, if a pin is unexpectedly stuck into an area of hysterical anaesthesia the patient does not flinch or wince. It has already been mentioned that hysterics are very suggestible, and the form their hysterical symptoms take is often subconsciously suggested to them by some preceding or underlying organic disease. In such cases a good deal of experience is needed in sorting out the organic from the hysterical symptoms, but this is often not very difficult, since the patient with a hysterical paralysis, for example, fails to show the physical signs of either an upper or a lower motor neurone lesion.

Fits are another manifestation of hysteria. The problem here is to distinguish them from epilepsy and it must be remembered that the same patient may at different times have both epileptic and hysterical fits. The latter, like every other hysterical symptom, are serving some subconscious purpose for the patient, and therefore he never has them when he is alone; they are always staged before a suitable audience. There is no orderly sequence of events, as in an epileptic fit; the patient shouts or screams and thrashes about with his limbs, but he avoids injuring himself, does not pass his water and shows no subsequent loss of reflexes. Furthermore, the fit may go on for very much longer than the epileptic variety—as long, in fact, as the suitable audience remains suitably impressed.

Treatment Dramatic relief of hysterical symptoms can often be achieved by making use of the abnormal suggestibility of the patient. This is done by firmly persuading him that his paralysis or whatever it may be has been cured and ordering him to use the limb or whatever function has been lost; such persuasion may be more effective if the patient is under hypnosis or is recovering from an anaesthetic given for the purpose. 'Miraculous' cures at Lourdes and elsewhere are usually of this type.

Before any such cure is attempted, however, it is important to consider very carefully the unhappy circumstances which have driven the patient into the refuge of hysterical illness. It has been known for a patient, dramatically relieved of his hysterical symptoms, to find the situation which caused them still present and to commit suicide. The first essential, therefore, is to ascertain what it is that the patient has found intolerable and if possible to put it right for him; in this task the psychiatric social worker (PSW) often plays an invaluable part. For many of life's difficulties, however, there is no cure, and where this applies it may be kinder in the long run to leave the patient with his hysterical illness.

Migraine

Patients subject to migraine are liable to recurrent attacks of sick headache, often accompanied by visual disturbances and other symptoms. The attacks usually start in adolescence and become less frequent and severe after middle age. Migrainous subjects are usually of an obsessional temperament and the attack frequently comes during the period of relaxation following a phase of intense activity or anxiety ('week-end migraine'). The symptoms are produced by spasm followed by dilatation in one or more of the intracranial arteries.

A typical attack starts with blurring of vision in one half of the visual field and in this area moving lights may be seen. After 20 minutes or so vision becomes normal again and the patient develops a severe headache, usually confined to one half of the head. The headache may last for many hours and the attack often terminates with nausea and vomiting.

Treatment In a few patients attacks seem to be precipitated by articles of diet, notably chocolate and citrus fruit, and it may be worth eliminating these for a test period. In others sudden exposure to bright lights or glare may start an attack; if so, care should be taken to avoid such exposure or to wear dark glasses. In most patients, however, no specific precipitant for attacks can be identified. Propranolol 10–20 mg t.d.s. or clonidine 0.025 mg t.d.s. are sometimes helpful in preventing attacks. For the attack itself soluble aspirin 600 mg with the anti-emetic metoclopromide (Maxolon) 10 mg may give adequate relief, but if not ergotamine tartrate 2 mg, either by mouth or as a suppository, may be tried. Although relieving headache ergotamine may make the sickness worse and as overdosage can lead to gangrene of the extremities it must always be given under careful medical supervision.

11

Diseases of the Skin

Eczema

There is a great deal of confusion about the meaning of the words 'eczema' and 'dermatitis', mainly due to the different senses in which these terms are used by different authorities. It is perhaps best to regard dermatitis as meaning any type of inflammation of the skin, and eczema as a particular variety of dermatitis characterised by a red, weeping eruption usually associated with itching, but some skin specialists make no such distinction and use the two words synonymously.

Some substances cause an eczematous reaction when applied to the skin of normal people; others do so only when applied to the skin of people who are specially sensitive. Less often eczema may result from the eating of particular foods. Infantile eczema occurs in babies who have inherited an abnormal tendency to develop hypersensitivity to foreign proteins, and these children frequently go on to suffer from hay fever, asthma and persistent patches of eczema in the flexures of the limbs.

Contact Eczema (or contact dermatitis) is extremely common. The substances which may cause eczema when applied to the skin are very numerous and may be classified into the following groups:

1 **Chemical.** Drugs are important members of this group. Almost any drug may cause eczema on the skin of a sensitive individual, but nurses should be particularly careful when giving injections of penicillin or streptomycin not to allow any of the solution to come in contact with their hands. Nickel (on suspender and brassiere clips), lipstick, nail varnish and hair dyes are common causes, and so are the dyes in furs and other articles of clothing. Soaps, bleaching agents and detergents constitute another big group.

2 **Substances of Plant Origin.** In this country the commonest plants to cause eczema are primulas and chrysanthemums.

3 **Micro-organisms.** Bacterial infections of the skin, such as impetigo or fungus infections, may be complicated by an eczematous reaction.

The **diagnosis** of contact eczema is usually suggested by the history of contact, and the site and distribution of the lesions and may be confirmed by a **patch test,** in which the suspected substance is applied to an area of normal skin, covered with a square of cellophane or jaconet and left for 24–48 hours. A positive result is the development within three or four days of an eczematous reaction in the area of skin covered.

Treatment of Eczema The most important point is the removal of the cause, if this is known. Thus avoidance of contact with the offending drug, dye, plant or whatever it may be, or change of work for patients with occupational eczema, is an obvious and usually effective remedy. Local symptomatic treatment has been immeasurably improved by the introduction of corticosteroid ointment, which may be combined with an antibiotic (as in the proprietary preparations 'Synalar N' and 'Betnovate N' cream).

Drug Eruptions

Drug eruptions are very common and may mimic the rashes of many other diseases, particularly measles and scarlet fever. There must be few drugs which never cause rashes, but the commonest offenders are the **barbiturates,** especially phenobarbitone, and the **sulphonamides. Streptomycin** is another common example; the other antituberculous drugs **PAS** and **isoniazid** also cause rashes, but less frequently. **Thiouracil** and **phenylbutazone** are other drugs worthy of special mention in this connection.

Iodides (usually taken in the form of potassium iodide in a cough mixture) occasionally cause remarkable large fungating, ulcerative lesions. The heavy metals **gold** and less often **arsenic** may cause a very severe generalised exfoliative dermatitis which is sometimes fatal. Nowadays **penicillin** rashes are among the commonest and most important. In a sensitised subject an injection of penicillin may cause an urticarial rash, angioneurotic oedema, or rarely death within a few minutes from anaphylaxis. This last complication occurs particularly in allergic people with a history of infantile eczema, hay fever and asthma; any such person who is known to have had a rash or any reaction following previous treatment with penicillin should on no account be given any more.

Treatment In mild cases withdrawal of the drug is all that is needed. At the other end of the scale, exfoliative dermatitis needs vigorous treatment with cortisone or ACTH, which must be continued in the lowest effective dosage until the rash has completely faded. When a heavy metal is the cause, the patient should also be given BAL (British antilewisite) intramuscularly, 3 mg per kg of body-weight every 6 hours for 3 days.

For anaphylactic shock following injection of a drug give an immediate injection of adrenaline 1:1000, 0.5 ml subcutaneously, after which it may be necessary for an intravenous infusion of plasma containing noradrenaline or aminophylline to be set up. A good rule is never to give a drug by injection without a solution of adrenaline ready for use if needed.

Infections of the Skin

Impetigo Contagiosa

This is an infection of the superficial layers of the skin with either streptococci or staphylococci, and it occurs mainly in dirty, neglected and debilitated children, sometimes as a complication of scabies or pediculosis. As the name implies, it is very infectious and it is spread either by direct contact or by the use of contaminated towels or clothes.

Clinical Features The first lesion is a pink macule up to half an inch in diameter, but within a few hours this becomes converted into first a superficial vesicle, then a pustule which quickly ruptures with the formation of a typical bright yellow crust. The face is the usual site. There is rarely any fever or constitutional disturbance.

Treatment Patients with severe infection should be given flucloxacillin (Floxapen) 250 mg 6-hourly by mouth. The essential local treatment is to remove the crusts with 1 per cent cetrimide (Savlon) or starch poultices. Antibiotic creams and lotions should be avoided because of the danger of sensitisation.

It is important to search for and treat any associated lesion, such as scabies or pediculosis capitis; the latter is particularly likely to be found in girls with long hair. The patient must of course be kept away from other children and must have his own towel and pillow-case, which should subsequently be sterilised by boiling.

Ringworm

This is a group of common fungus infections of the skin which affect mainly the scalp, the groin and the feet.

Tinea Capitis (ringworm of the scalp)

This infection is seen mainly in children under 10, particularly boys, and never persists beyond adolescence. The scalp shows a number of rounded or oval patches which are covered with fine greyish-white scales and from which most of the hairs have fallen out. The ringworm fungus fluoresces a bright green colour under Wood's light, and this examination is therefore helpful in diagnosis. The fungus can also be identified microscopically in stumps of hair removed from one of the patches.

Treatment Griseofulvin 250 mg by mouth four times daily for a month or longer is now the treatment of choice. This is usually a very effective drug (and one which causes few side-effects), but older methods of treatment are still occasionally needed for recurrent or refractory cases. Repeated daily applications of Whitfield's ointment to the scalp followed by vigorous shampooing may be tried; but in some children well below the age of puberty the only effective therapy is the application of X-rays to the scalp in sufficient dosage to cause all the hair to fall out in the next two or three weeks.

Tinea Cruris (fungus infection in the groin)

This infection occurs mainly in young adults, particularly men, and may be acquired either by direct contact or from infected clothing or articles such as lavatory seats. It causes a red, slightly raised patch extending from the crutch for two or three inches down the inner aspect of each thigh. There is sometimes itching in the affected area. The infection is seen mainly in hot weather and is more common therefore in the tropics.

Treatment Whitfield's ointment is usually very effective, but relapses in subsequent spells of hot weather are common.

Tinea Pedis (*fungus infection of the foot; athlete's foot*)

This infection occurs in two forms, one causing vesicles and subsequent desquamation on the sole of the foot, and the other causing fissuring and maceration of the skin in the clefts between the toes. Like tinea cruris, with which it may be associated, this infection is seen mainly in young adults and is acquired from the floors of public baths or changing-rooms.

Treatment Whitfield's ointment, Castellani's paint and undecylenic acid ointment are three among a number of effective remedies. Relapse is common, however, and to try to prevent it careful attention to the hygiene of the feet is important. The feet should be washed daily, carefully dried and powdered and the socks should be changed every day.

Parasitic Diseases

Scabies

The animal causing scabies is a mite (*Sarcoptes scabiei hominis*). It has four pairs of legs, and the female, which causes the trouble, is about 0.3 mm long, being therefore just visible to the naked eye; the male is smaller. The female makes a burrow up to a centimetre in length in the superficial layers of the skin and lays about 30 to 40 eggs in it. Each egg hatches out in 4 to 8 days into a larval form which leaves the burrow and eventually matures into the adult form.

Infection is mainly acquired by sleeping with an infected person. It may therefore be a venereal infection, or children may contract it as a result of sharing their parents' bed or from each other. Less often, infected blankets, bedding or clothes may transmit the infection.

Clinical Features The burrow is the characteristic lesion of scabies and appears as a fine, often zig-zag, hair-like line in the epidermis, greyish or whitish in colour and 0.5 – 1 cm in length. At the far end a tiny pinhead vesicle may be seen. These burrows occur mainly in the webs and sides of the fingers, the ulnar sides of the hands, the anterior axillary folds, the lower abdomen and penis, and the lower part of the buttocks. They cause intense itching, particularly when the patient is warm in bed. As a result of scratching, secondary infection is common, and there may be an extensive papular and pustular eruption.

Diagnosis is usually easy from the history of intense itching and the discovery of the typical burrows, and may be confirmed by the identification of the female acarus or its eggs in a microscopical preparation of scrapings from a burrow.

Treatment This starts with a hot bath, the patient being instructed to scrub with a nail-brush and soap all areas where there are burrows. After drying himself, the patient is painted from head to foot with a solution consisting of equal parts of benzyl benzoate, soft soap and industrial spirit, sparing only the head and neck, which are never affected by scabies. After the solution has dried, another coat of it is applied. Next morning the lotion is applied again and allowed to dry before the patient dresses. That night another hot bath is taken to wash off the remains of the benzyl benzoate solution and a complete change of clothing and bed linen is made. Gloves and other articles which are difficult to disinfest should be laid aside for 3 weeks, at the end of which time all acari they contain will have died.

It need hardly be said that all contacts with the patient, parricularly those within his own family circle, should be treated at the same time to prevent reinfection.

Lice

These are blood-sucking parasites which mainly infest hairy parts of the body. The female produces several hundred eggs, each of which is attached to a hair and is commonly known as a nit. A larva is hatched out from the egg in 6–9 days and develops into a mature louse in 1–2 weeks.

Pediculosis Capitis (infestation with head lice)

The louse concerned is *Pediculus humanus capitis*, which is about 3 mm long and 1 mm broad. It infests the scalp, the nits being attached mainly to hairs at the back and sides of the head. Since the louse deposits the eggs on hairs close to the scalp, and since they have hatched out by the time the hair has grown an inch or two, the search for nits should be concentrated on the hair close to the head.

The diagnosis depends usually on the discovery of nits, since the lice themselves are few in number and difficult to find. Nits are greyish-white, oval, shiny, opalescent structures firmly attached to the hairs.

Infection is acquired by direct transmission from person to person or by wearing infected headgear; and since the lice flourish particularly in long hair which is seldom washed, infestation occurs mainly in women and girls living under poor hygienic conditions. Patients recently infected usually complain of irritation of the scalp, but those who have had head lice for a long time often seem to suffer no inconvenience at all. When there has been much scratching, septic lesions of the scalp are a common complication.

Treatment Gamma benzene hexachloride application is effective but may have to be repeated after a week. The hair should be shampooed 12 hours after the application and combed while wet with a fine-toothed comb. It is much easier to treat short hair.

Pediculosis Corporis (infestation with body lice)

Pediculus humanus corporis is similar to the head louse but slightly bigger. It normally lives in the clothes, and deposits its eggs in the seams and folds of woollen undergarments.

Clinical Features Infestation causes a variable amount of itching; scratch-marks are seen mainly around the shoulders, buttocks and the front of the thighs, and there may be a widespread eruption from secondary bacterial infection in these situations. Tramps and vagrants after lifelong infestation may develop a generalised pigmentation of the skin like that seen in Addison's disease ('vagabond's pigmentation').

The diagnosis is established by discovery of the louse or its ova in the seams of the patient's underclothes.

Treatment Gamma benzene hexachloride is applied as a 0.6% dusting powder and scrubbed on to infected hairy areas as a 2% lotion in a detergent base. Underclothes must be washed and ironed and bedding and other clothing autoclaved. After treatment the patient takes a hot bath and puts on clean clothes.

In addition to their direct effects, infestation with head and body lice is important in the spread of typhus and relapsing fevers.

'Pediculosis' Pubis (infestation with 'crab' lice)

This louse is not in fact of the species *Pediculus*, its scientific name being *Phthirius pubis*. Its life-history is, however, similar to that of the pediculi, but it is smaller (about 2 mm by 1.5 mm) and does not spread typhus or any other disease.

Clinical Features It infests particularly the pubic region, though in very hairy men the whole of the trunk, the thighs and upper arms may be involved. On close inspection the adult lice can be seen, lying flat on the skin and holding on to a hair at each side; the eggs are very similar to the nits of *Pediculus humanus* and are closely attached to the coarser body-hairs.

Infection is acquired mainly by sexual intercourse, and is therefore seen most frequently in young adults.

Treatment is as for *Pediculosis corporis*.

General Management of Patients with Skin Diseases

Most patients with skin diseases are treated in the outpatient department or by their own doctor, and only if the condition is severe are they admitted to hospital. The tendency is to regard skin diseases as incurable, but in fact the great majority will respond to treatment if it is carried out regularly and conscientiously.

Treatment is usually done by the patient himself, and his co-operation is essential. The constant attention needed often becomes irksome, however, and takes a great deal of time, and if the patient is unable to carry out his own treatment he may have to be admitted to hospital.

Nurses caring for such a patient must appreciate how upsetting it is to be disfigured by a skin disease and that he may be very sensitive about his condition. Tact, understanding and kindness must be shown at all times. The nurse may feel somewhat repulsed, but at no time must the patient be allowed to sense this. Very few skin diseases are infectious.

When preparations likely to stain linen are being applied, the patient should be warned to use old underclothes and sheets which can be discarded subsequently.

In treating any skin condition it is important to relieve irritation and pain, to prevent scratching and to improve the patient's general health.

Irritation can be relieved by the use of soothing applications which will vary according to the type of lesion; antihistamine drugs such as phenergan given orally or anthisan cream applied to the skin will usually give relief. The diet must not include stimulating highly-seasoned foods and all drinks should be cool. Non-irritating clothing must be next to the skin and overheated rooms must be avoided. A sensitive skin should always be protected from direct rays of the sun. It is often necessary to restrain children by applying covered cardboard splints to the arms. Tube gauze bandage may also be useful and does not limit movement. Splinting for adults may be necessary at night, as they may scratch the skin during sleep.

Pain is usually relieved by the type of external application used. Dressings must be done as often as necessary and should not be allowed to become dry and uncomfortable. Sleep is important and chloral hydrate is probably the most suitable hypnotic. Sedatives such as phenobarbitone may be ordered.

Diet A non-stimulating diet has already been mentioned. When dietary factors are suspected to be the cause of the condition, great care must be taken to note any reactions when new foods are added to the diet. A well-balanced diet is necessary; a high protein content is usually given for tissue repair and the carbohydrate content should be reduced. Vitamins may be given in tablet form and plenty of fluids should be taken.

Bowels Constipation is to be avoided.

Urine Examination of the urine is necessary in certain cases, particularly if the skin disease is due to streptococcal infection which may be complicated by nephritis.

Local Applications

The drugs used in the treatment of skin diseases are many and varied and include antibiotics, chemical preparations, aniline dyes, heavy metals, alkalis, coal tar and, more recently, cortisone. It is, however, important to remember that such drugs may be made up in any type of base, for example, in a lotion, cream, ointment or powder. The choice of base depends on its suitability for the particular type of skin eruption and will be changed as the lesions change.

Cleansing Agents Cetavlon is now widely used for cleaning almost any type of lesion. Boracic and starch poultice, well made and applied, is probably the most effective method of softening and removing crusts. Medicated baths given at a temperature of 37.2°C are both soothing and cleansing. To 10–11 litres of water may be added 66 g of sodium chloride (making normal saline), or 96 g of bran or oatmeal in a muslin bag; or crystals of potassium permanganate sufficient to colour the water a pale pink. Olive oil or cetavlon are useful for removing old paste or ointment.

Powders Zinc oxide, zinc carbonate, starch and boric powder will protect the skin from external irritation. They should only be applied to dry surfaces, for if there is exudation the powder cakes and becomes hard, causing irritation.

Lotions Simple aqueous solutions of active drugs such as zinc sulphate are applied as wet dressings; they should be covered by a protective tissue and renewed 3- to 4-hourly. In powdery lotions the drug is insoluble and suspended in water and glycerine; calamine (zinc carbonate) is often used in this form. The bottle must be well shaken and the lotion may be dabbed on with cotton wool or painted on with a brush. The water evaporates, leaving the powder on the skin. Lotions may be used for any erythematous and papular eruption and are very useful in conditions where exudation is profuse.

Varnishes Varnishes are liquid preparations (acetone being used as the solvent) which when painted on the skin leave a thin covering. The aniline dyes are often used as varnishes, for example an aqueous solution of 1 per cent gentian violet. They are useful for small pustular eruptions.

Ointments Ointments are commonly used. Purified paraffin molle is very useful. Animal fats (lard) or vegetable oils such as olive oil or almond oil may be used with wax and will rub into the skin more readily. These form the base of the cold creams. They are used when there is dryness or scaling of the skin, but are avoided when exudation is present.

Pastes Pastes contain a high percentage of a powder with an animal or mineral ointment and are applied spread on calico or linen. Ichthyol paste is commonly used.

Creams Creams are thin emulsions of water and oil in which an insoluble powder is suspended; calamine cream is an example. They may be rubbed into the skin or spread on material before application.

Steroid Therapy has revolutionised the treatment of many skin diseases, notably pemphigus. Prednisolone tablets may be given orally or more often hydrocortisone ointment is applied locally. Adequate dosage and gradual withdrawal are of great importance, and observations of weight and blood pressure must be made regularly when the drug is being given by mouth.

12

Infectious Diseases

Definition Although the term 'infectious disease' might logically be applied to any illness which results from invasion of the body by a micro-organism, its use is customarily restricted to those diseases which spread by direct contact from person to person. In this chapter, therefore, we shall not be concerned with diseases like pneumonia or bacterial endocarditis, which, though due to infection, can safely be nursed in general wards without special barrier precautions.

Infection and Immunity

The result of any infection depends partly on the virulence and numbers of the invading organisms and partly on the state of the patient's defences against them. The state of the defences depends on two factors: the degree of natural immunity inherited from the parents, which may be reduced by such general influences as malnutrition, worry and overwork; and whether there is any acquired immunity resulting from previous infection with this particular organism. Most infectious diseases confer lifelong specific immunity, so that second attacks are very unusual. Furthermore, suitable injections of killed or weakened organisms or their toxins may stimulate this specific immunity without actively causing any clinical illness; this fact is the basis of the immunisation procedures which are so important in the prevention of diseases such as diphtheria, tetanus and typhoid. **Passive immunisation** means conferring temporary protection against a disease by injecting serum which has been taken from someone with an active immunity and which therefore contains a high concentration of specific antibodies.

Carriers Some people who are themselves immune from a particular infectious disease may nevertheless harbour the specific organisms and transmit them from time to time to susceptible persons, either by direct contact or by infecting food or water. This carrier state is particularly important in the spread of typhoid fever.

Routes of Infection The invading organism usually gains access to the patient either in inspired air ('droplet infection') or in contaminated food or drink.

Incubation Period After gaining access to the tissues of a susceptible individual, the invading organisms take some time to multiply and consolidate their position before the symptoms of the disease appear. This interval is known as the incubation period. Its duration varies widely in the different infectious diseases, but remains fairly constant in each of them. The approximate length of the incubation period of common specific fevers is:

Less than 7 days	Diphtheria
	Scarlet fever
10 to 14 days	Measles
	Whooping cough
	Smallpox
	Enteric fever
14 to 21 days	Chickenpox
(usually nearer 21)	German measles
	Mumps

It is important to know the incubation period of the various specific fevers, since it is occasionally helpful in diagnosis if the date of exposure to infection is known and also because it enables one to forecast the possible appearance of the disease in people who have been in contact with the original patient. For a serious disease such as smallpox it may be advisable to isolate such contacts until it is known whether or not they have contracted the disease; the duration of this quarantine is worked out by adding a few days (to be on the safe side) to the known incubation period.

Stage of Invasion At the end of the incubation period the infecting organism or its toxic products become distributed throughout the body and give rise to the symptoms and signs of the disease. Common to all infectious diseases are fever, headache, general malaise, loss of appetite, dry furred tongue, hot dry skin and scanty highly-concentrated urine; but in addition each has special features, which in many of them include a typical rash, which enable the diagnosis to be made.

Scheme of Prophylactic Inoculations for Children

Age		*Vaccine*	*Dose*
3 months	(1)	'Triple vaccine' (against diphtheria, whooping cough and tetanus)	0.5 ml
	(2)	Oral polio vaccine	3 drops (on a lump of sugar)
4 months	(1)	'Triple vaccine'	0.5 ml
	(2)	Polio vaccine	3 drops
5 months	(1)	'Triple vaccine'	0.5 ml
	(2)	Polio vaccine	3 drops
12 months		Measles vaccine	0.5 ml
17 months		'Triple vaccine'	0.5 ml
$4\frac{1}{2}$ years	(1)	Combined adsorbed diphtheria vaccine and tetanus toxoid	0.5 ml
	(2)	Polio vaccine	3 drops

Routine vaccination of children against smallpox is no longer recommended in the UK since the risk of contracting the disease is now less than the risk of developing a serious complication of vaccination.

Encephalopathy is a rare complication of whooping cough vaccination and is more likely to occur in infants with a history of convulsions; such children should be given combined diphtheria and tetanus vaccine instead of triple vaccine. Children with a history of asthma, hay fever or eczema have a high incidence of allergic reactions after injections; they must therefore be kept under observation for half an hour after inoculations and adrenaline must be immediately available for injection if needed. When a severe local reaction occurs after the first injection of triple vaccine it is probably the whooping cough component which is responsible and for the subsequent injections it may be advisable to use only the combined diphtheria and tetanus vaccine.

General Nursing Precautions for Care of Infectious Diseases

As far as possible the nurse caring for a patient with an infectious disease should be known to be immune to it. Thus before nursing a case of smallpox she must have had a recent successful vaccination;

for enteric she should have had TAB inoculations; for diphtheria she should be Schick negative; and for tuberculosis she should be Mantoux positive. The health record of each nurse should include particulars of the infectious diseases she has had, as well as the results of Schick, Mantoux and other tests and details of any active immunisation procedure. The nurse must look after her own general health with particular attention to regular meals, adequate number of hours of sleep and fresh air off duty.

The object of the precautions adopted in the nursing of infectious diseases is to limit the spread of infection, and this is achieved by isolating the patient. Whether in a special hospital, a general hospital or at home, the basic principles of isolation are the same and the most conscientious nursing care is required.

Barrier Nursing

The technique is known as 'barrier' nursing, and every patient known or suspected to be suffering from an infectious disease is isolated in this way. The first principle is to provide a 'barrier' round the patient to prevent direct transmission of the organisms to other patients; this is done by increasing the space between the beds in the ward or by using a cubicle or separate room. Secondly, to prevent indirect transmission of infection the patient's cutlery, crockery and linen are kept separate, everything which has been near him being considered a possible source of infection.

When patients are nursed in an open ward a screen placed at the foot of the bed serves as a reminder that barrier precautions are being observed. Gowns are provided for all medical and nursing staff who are attending the patients. The gowns may be hung within the 'barrier' with the 'dirty' side outermost; if hung outside the barrier the 'dirty' side must be turned inwards. In this way contamination of ordinary clothing is prevented, but the technique of putting on and removing gowns requires great care. The hands must be washed before removing the gown and again after leaving the barrier.

All utensils should either be clearly marked and be kept separate or, if facilities are available, sterilised and stored in the usual manner. If available disposable utensils should be used.

To prevent the spread of infection it is important to know how the infection is transmitted, so that the particular route of infection can be blocked. For example, the attendant must take particular care to wear a mask if there is droplet infection, but if the source of infection is faeces and urine the emphasis will be on disposal of excreta and washing of hands. It is important to bear in mind that the commonest way for infection to spread is by the hands; special consideration should therefore be given to the method of disposal of materials infected by excreta or discharges and to cleanliness of the hands.

Disposal of Infectious Material Excreta should be completely covered with disinfectant, e.g. formalin 1–250 for half an hour, and then disposed of in the usual way. Linen fouled with infectious excreta should also be soaked in the above solution before being laundered. Bedpans and urinals are kept separate or boiled each time after use.

Secretions and Discharges Paper handkerchiefs and dressing swabs contaminated by infectious discharges should be dropped immediately into a paper bag, which after the top has been screwed up is dropped into a container for incineration. Infectious linen should be placed in a specially labelled bag to send to the laundry.

Masks Disposable masks are a protection, but unless used with care they can be a danger. The mask must be worn over the nostrils and mouth, and it must be remembered that the outside may be infected and must not be touched. When removed after use it is held by the strings and dropped into a covered receptacle kept for the purpose. Where disposable utensils and gowns are available, the routine is simplified.

Care of Hands Nurses, doctors, medical students and others should thoroughly wash their hands after attending the patient and again on leaving the ward, and of course before meals. Careful drying is important, after which hand cream should be applied. Preferably paper towels should be used and discarded, or an adequate supply of clean towels should be available.

Bacterial Infections

Diphtheria

Diphtheria is an infection of the throat, nose or larynx (or occasionally the skin), and although the organism, *Corynebacterium diphtheriae*, remains localised at this site, it produces a very powerful poison or exotoxin which becomes widely distributed and may cause serious or even fatal effects on other parts of the body. The amount of exotoxin produced by different strains of the organism varies a good deal, and this is one reason why some patients are much more severely ill than others. The other reason for the variation in severity is the state of immunity of the patient at the time he acquires the infection.

Immunity Immunity to diphtheria may be acquired in three ways:

(1) After recovery from an attack of the disease.

(2) After repeated subclinical infection, that is, as a result of coming in contact from time to time with organisms insufficient in either numbers or virulence to cause a full-scale attack of diphtheria.

(3) As a result of active immunisation by inoculation. It is because of the widespread inoculation of children that this killing disease is now much less common than it used to be, but this is no reason for complacency; if all children were immunised there would be no deaths from diphtheria.

Patients who have acquired an active immunity in one of these three ways are very unlikely to contract diphtheria, and if they do the illness is a mild one without serious complications.

The Schick Test is used to detect whether or not an individual has immunity against diphtheria, that is, whether he can produce an antitoxin to neutralise the exotoxin of diphtheria. Diphtheria toxin 0.2 ml is injected into the skin of the left forearm, and 0.2 ml of the same toxin which has been heated to 70°C to destroy its potency is injected into the skin of the right forearm to act as a control. The result is read in 5–7 days, as follows:

Positive. An area of redness and swelling at the site of injection on the left arm, with no reaction on the right (control) arm. This indicates that the person tested has no antitoxin with which to neutralise the toxin injected; in other words, he is **susceptible** to diphtheria.

Negative. No reaction in either arm. The injected toxin has been neutralised by antitoxin and the subject is therefore **immune** to diphtheria.

Positive plus 'Pseudo Reaction'. There is redness and swelling on both arms, but more on the left (test) arm than on the right (control) arm. The reaction on the right arm and part of the reaction on the left are due to some factor in the injections other than the actual toxin; the extra reaction on the left must be due to unneutralised toxin and the subject is therefore **susceptible** to diphtheria.

Negative plus 'Pseudo Reaction'. There is equal redness and swelling on both arms: the subject is immune to diphtheria.

Active Immunisation All children should be immunised against diphtheria. The Schick test is used on adults who are exposed to special risk of infection, for example nurses and medical students, and those shown to be susceptible are immunised.

Immunisation of children is effected by three injections of alum precipitated toxoid (APT). The first dose of 0.3–0.5 ml is given between 3 and 9 months, the second of 0.5 ml is given 4 weeks later and the final 'boosting' dose of 0.2 ml at the age of four.

Adults are immunised in the same way, but if the preliminary Schick test shows a 'positive plus pseudo' result unpleasant reactions may follow the use of APT, and it is better to use toxoid antitoxin floccules (TAF). This is given in three doses of 1 ml each at intervals of 2 weeks and rarely causes any side-effects.

Clinical Features of Diphtheria Diphtheria is classified clinically according to the exact site of infection. The commonest variety is **faucial** diphtheria, in which the characteristic membrane of the disease forms in the throat. There is a short incubation of only 3 or 4 days from exposure to infection. Points which help to distinguish diphtheria from streptococcal tonsillitis are:

(1) The throat is not so sore and the temperature usually not so high, but the general exhaustion and 'toxaemia' are much greater.

(2) The lymph-nodes in the neck are usually enlarged to a greater extent, in severe cases causing a collar of swelling sometimes referred to as the 'bull-neck'.

(3) The exudate in the throat is not confined to yellowish spots on the tonsils, but forms a continuous greyish sheet of membrane which often extends forward over the soft palate and backwards on to the pharyngeal wall and is so firmly adherent that any attempt to wipe it off leaves a bleeding surface.

Less common and more difficult to diagnose are **nasal diphtheria,** in which the membrane is confined to the nose, where it may lead to a bloodstained nasal discharge; and **laryngeal diphtheria,** a very dangerous form in which the membrane on the larynx may obstruct breathing and necessitate emergency tracheotomy.

Cutaneous Diphtheria is very rare in this country, but during the War was a common cause of so-called 'jungle sores' or 'desert sores', the true nature of which was often not realised until the development of some postdiphtheritic complication.

Complications The complications of diphtheria are due to the effect on the heart and nervous system of the toxin absorbed from the lesions in the upper respiratory tract.

Carditis may occur at the height of the infection and is characterised by vomiting, greyish pallor, weak rapid pulse, low blood pressure, diminished urinary output, usually with some albuminuria, and sometimes pain over the heart. Sudden death is not uncommon in these cases.

Paralysis. Paralysis of the palate is the commonest type, and causes a nasal voice and regurgitation of food through the nose. It usually appears in the second or third weeks and may extend to the pharyngeal muscles, causing difficulty in swallowing; or rarely to the intercostal muscles or diaphragm, causing weakness in breathing and necessitating treatment in a mechanical respirator. There is sometimes paralysis of the ciliary muscle in the eye, causing difficulty in reading. Towards the fifth or sixth weeks peripheral neuritis may occur, causing weakness in the limbs which eventually clears up completely: it is this complication which may lead to the recognition of diphtheritic sores on the skin.

Treatment Although a throat (or nasal) swab should always be taken whenever diphtheria is suspected, the disease is so dangerous that treatment must invariably be started at once without waiting for the result of the culture.

The most important measure is the immediate administration of antitoxin. The dose varies from about 8000–100 000 units, according to the severity of the infection, and it is usual to give half the total dose intramuscularly and then if there has been no serum reaction within 15–30 minutes to give the remainder intravenously. If a serum reaction such as vomiting, wheezing or collapse occurs, an immediate subcutaneous injection of 1/1000 adrenaline 0.5 ml must be given, and on no account must any serum be administered intravenously, owing to the serious risk of death from anaphylactic shock. It is usual also to give penicillin, 100 000–500 000 units every 4 hours, but it should be stressed that this is less important than the antitoxin.

Nursing Care Diphtheria is moderately infectious and spreads usually by droplet infection. Outbreaks can sometimes be traced to a convalescent carrier. Discharges from the nose and throat are infectious and may contaminate fomites.

The patient must be strictly isolated and kept in a warm and even temperature. He tends to feel cold because of the lowered blood pressure, and warm blankets will be required next to him. Absolute rest is vital, to prevent any unnecessary strain on the heart muscle. He is nursed in a recumbent position, with a flat pillow under his head; he may have to be kept in this position for several weeks, before gradually being propped up with one extra pillow at a time on the instructions of the doctor. Due to the severe toxaemia, the patient is very pale, listless and disinterested in his surroundings and has a fast weak pulse.

The nurse must do everything for him. Two nurses are required for giving bedpans and care of pressure areas. He must be handled gently and smoothly and sudden movement or activity on the part of the patient should be prevented. Bathing is reduced to the minimum, face, hands and back being washed only twice a day in the early stages. Local treatment of the throat probably does more harm than good, but ordinary cleanliness of the mouth is important. Lanoline should be applied to the lips to prevent soreness.

A simple enema will cause least upset to the patient, but this need only be given every three days in the acute stage. Lubricants such as liquid paraffin can be given daily.

The diet must be light and nourishing and glucose should be added to all drinks. Great care is required when feeding the patient, particularly in the case of young children, who find it difficult to feed when lying down and who tend to choke when drinking. If palatal and pharyngeal paralysis are present, tube-feeding will be necessary.

Adequate sleep and rest are essential and constant vigilance is necessary for early recognition of any complications (p. 000). In the early convalescent stage activities must be gradually increased and strictly regulated.

Laryngeal diphtheria is seen mainly in infants and young children. Obstruction may occur rapidly, and manifests itself by persistent restlessness, an anxious expression, inspiration becoming increasingly difficult until stridor develops and all accessory muscles of respiration are being used. There is obvious sucking in of the soft parts of the chest wall on inspiration. Emergency tracheotomy must be performed without delay if the child becomes cyanosed.

Prevention When a case of diphtheria occurs in a closed community such as a school or a hospital ward combined active and passive immunisation of the contacts should be carried out. Antitoxin 1000 units is given into the deltoid of one arm and the first 0.5 ml of APT into the other. Four weeks later the second 0.5 ml APT completes the procedure.

Sometimes an outbreak of diphtheria can be traced to a healthy 'carrier', and it is important that his infection be eradicated to prevent further spread of the disease. This can sometimes be achieved by giving large doses of penicillin, 2–4 million units daily, combined with sulphadimidine 4–6 g daily for up to a week. If the infection persists some surgical procedure such as tonsillectomy may be indicated.

Whooping Cough (Pertussis)

Whooping cough is an infection of the respiratory tract by *Bordetella pertussis*. In this country at present it is the most serious of the acute specific fevers of childhood, not only causing many deaths in young children, particularly under the age of 12 months, but also occasionally leading to serious damage to the bronchi and lungs (see bronchiectasis, p. 56).

Clinical Features After an incubation period of 7–14 days the child develops what is thought at first to be an ordinary cold in the head, but within about a week of the onset the paroxysms of coughing have usually become so severe and typical that the true diagnosis is obvious. A characteristic paroxysm consists of a deep inspiration followed by a rapid series of explosive coughs during expiration. This sequence of events is practically diagnostic of whooping cough. In some, but not all, cases the paroxysm ends with the inspiration of air through a partially closed glottis causing the classical 'whoop', and very frequently, too, the bout of coughing leads to vomiting.

The preliminary catarrhal stage is short in duration but highly infectious; the paroxysmal coughing and whooping may continue for many weeks, but the infectivity is now very slight.

Complications Broncho-pneumonia is the most serious complication and is responsible for most of the deaths which occur in infancy. Collapse of one or more segments of the lung from plugging of the bronchi or bronchioles by sticky mucus may lead eventually to bronchiectasis. Otitis media is the other common infective complication. When the paroxysms of coughing are severe, subconjunctival haemorrhage may occur, and an ulcer may form under the tongue from abrasion against the lower incisor teeth; no treatment is required for either of these traumatic lesions. Finally, convulsions occur more often in whooping cough than in any other of the specific fevers.

Treatment It is doubtful if whooping cough responds to any antibiotic. Claims have been made for aureomycin and chloramphenicol, however, and it is probably wise to give a course of one of these if only to reduce the risk of secondary infection by other organisms. The dose is 250 mg 6-hourly for five to seven days.

Nursing Care Whooping cough is not highly infectious. Spread occurs by droplet, but close contact is necessary, for example, between children in a family.

The patient should be isolated from other children as early as possible, since the disease is at its most infectious during the first few days. Only when home conditions are unfavourable or the child's general health is poor is he likely to be nursed in hospital.

The patient should be in bed in a well-ventilated room. He will be sitting up and protected from chills and draughts by warm clothing. When the temperature is normal he may be allowed up, and will be able to go out quite soon if the weather is suitable, but he must be kept away from other children for three or four weeks. During a paroxysm someone should go to the child at once to reassure and comfort him.

A nourishing diet is important; at first fluids and soft foods are preferable, as dry and more solid food tends to cause coughing. If the paroxysms cause vomiting, the child becomes frightened of eating, and a good deal of coaxing will be necessary. Food may be accepted more readily if given immediately after vomiting has occurred.

In infants vomiting can be a serious complication. Diarrhoea may often be present, too, and they rapidly suffer from loss of body fluids. Parenteral fluids may have to be given. At this age careful observations for signs of broncho-pneumonia must be made. When the paroxysms occur the baby should be lifted up at once; if they are severe, oxygen inhalations may be necessary following the paroxysms. Cough depressants and a belladonna mixture may be given to relieve the cough and relax spasm.

After three to four weeks there is little danger of infection, although the cough may persist for months. Children living in towns should have a holiday by the sea or in the country to give them every opportunity to build up their resistance to respiratory infections. Malt and cod liver oil are beneficial and a course of ultraviolet light may help.

Prevention This is done by giving three injections of combined diphtheria, tetanus and pertussis vaccine at 6 months, 8 months and 12 months.

Scarlet Fever

When seen in historical perspective many infective diseases go through periods of increased or decreased severity, and scarlet fever at the present time is a much less serious illness than it was in the first two decades of this century. It is a haemolytic streptococcal infection which is distinguished from other diseases due to the same organism by its typical rash; this rash indicates that the streptococcus concerned is of a strain which produces a special erythrogenic (literally 'red-making') toxin and that the patient is susceptible to its action.

The Dick Test can be used to demonstrate immunity or susceptibility to the erythrogenic toxin. 0.2 ml of toxin is injected into the skin of the forearm, no control injection in the other arm being necessary. A red swollen area at the site of injection in 24 hours shows that the person tested is **susceptible** (Dick positive); no reaction shows that he is immune (Dick negative).

Clinical Features After a short incubation period of less than a week the illness starts abruptly with sore throat, fever, shivering and frequently vomiting. Small children often do not complain of sore throat, but on examination the tonsils and fauces are very red and swollen and the tonsils may be covered with patches of soft, yellowish exudate. At first the tongue is covered with a white fur, which peels off from the edges during the next two or three days, leaving a clean surface with enlarged red papillae—the 'strawberry' or 'raspberry' tongue.

The **rash** appears on the second day, and is described as a punctate erythema; the skin is a bright scarlet colour, and on close inspection is seen to be covered with minute red spots. It appears first behind the ears and on the side of the neck and spreads rapidly over the whole body, but avoiding the area round the mouth (giving the so-called 'circumoral pallor') and tending to be particularly heavy in flexures such as the axillae, cubital fossae and groins. After about a week 'pin-hole desquamation' of the skin starts: little round pieces of dead skin flake off, temporarily leaving small holes in the superficial layers of the epidermis.

Complications are relatively uncommon nowadays, but spread of the infection may occur in weakly children to cause otitis media, sinusitis, suppurating lymph-nodes in the neck, bronchopneumonia or septicaemia. Perhaps the most important complication is **acute nephritis** (p. 107), which does not develop until two or three weeks after the scarlet fever has subsided.

Treatment For the mildest form of the disease oral penicillin (phenoxymethyl penicillin) 250 mg four times daily is satisfactory. More severely ill patients should be given IM benzyl penicillin 0.5–1.0 mega units 6-hourly for 2 days, followed by oral penicillin. Patients allergic to penicillin may be given erythromycin 250–500 mg orally every 6 hours for 10 days.

Enteric Fever

Enteric is the name applied to a group of diseases which consists of typhoid fever and paratyphoid A, B and C. These are due to closely related salmonella organisms and are very similar clinically, though true typhoid tends to be more serious and has a higher mortality. Typhoid and paratyphoid B occur all over the world, the latter being the commonest of the enteric fevers in this country; paratyphoid A is found mainly in the East; paratyphoid C is rare.

One of the bacteriological characteristics of the salmonella organisms, of which the enteric members are a subgroup, is inability to ferment lactose; the preliminary report from the laboratory, therefore, on cultures from patients with typhoid or paratyphoid often refers to 'non-lactose fermenters which are being further investigated'.

Method of Spread Enteric fever is spread by contamination of food or water by excreta from carriers or from patients with the disease. It is therefore prevalent in countries whose standards of sanitation are low and the sharp reduction in its incidence in this country at the end of the nineteenth century was due to the provision of methods of sewage disposal which prevent access to the water supplies. In countries with good sanitation outbreaks can usually be traced to unsuspecting carriers of the disease who are engaged in the handling of foodstuffs.

Clinical Features After an incubation period of about a fortnight there is usually a gradual onset of headache, aching in the limbs, tiredness, cough and fever, which typically rises in 'step-ladder fashion' by about half a degree (C) each day to reach a height of perhaps 40°C towards the end of the first week. For the next week, or sometimes much longer, the temperature continues at this high level, showing very little variation throughout the 24 hours. The pulse usually does not show the increase in rate which accompanies most febrile illnesses, often remaining between 70 and 80 per minute through the whole course of the disease.

In suspected cases careful watch must be kept about the end of the first week for the appearance of the characteristic rash. This often consists of no more than a few 'rose-spots', which can easily be overlooked, but which nevertheless are very typical of the disease. They occur particularly on the abdomen or chest, and appear for a few days in a succession of small 'crops' of tiny pink spots, each not more than 1–2 mm in diameter and each one lasting for only 24 hours or so. It is useful, therefore, to make a ring round each spot seen, so that next day if any new ones have appeared it is clear at a glance that they are a new crop. The spleen often becomes palpable at about the same time as the rash appears.

Most patients are constipated during the first few days, but towards the end of the second week the abdomen becomes distended and diarrhoea sets in. By this time if the attack is a severe one the patient is very gravely ill and may pass into the 'typhoid state', in which he remains throughout the 24 hours in what has been called a 'coma-vigil': drowsy and confused, but continually muttering to himself, plucking at the bedclothes and groping for non-existent objects. The faeces are now fluid and light yellow in colour ('pea-soup stools') and up to 20 may be passed in 24 hours.

Gradual improvement usually occurs during the third or fourth weeks; the temperature slowly subsides to normal over a period of several days, the diarrhoea stops, the mind becomes clearer and the other symptoms also slowly disappear.

Diagnostic Investigations (a) **Blood Culture** is by far the best way of establishing the diagnosis, and as the organisms circulate in the blood only during the first week, it is extremely important that blood should be taken for culture as early as possible, preferably during the first three days.

(b) **Agglutinations (Widal Test).** Agglutinins are antibodies which appear in the blood in response to the infection, their concentration increasing as the disease progresses. Therefore, if the sample of blood taken during the second week contains a higher 'titre' (i.e., concentration) of typhoid agglutinins than the sample taken during the first week, this may be taken as evidence that the patient has typhoid fever.

Culture of faeces and urine is not of much value for diagnosis, since the organisms are not usually excreted by the bowel and kidneys until about the third week of the disease. Such cultures should always be taken during convalescence, however, to make sure that the patient does not continue as a persistent 'carrier' of the disease. In such cases it is usually the faecal culture which remains positive, and as the organisms may have settled down in the gall bladder, passing down into the intestine in the bile, cholecystectomy may be necessary to prevent the patient being a continual menace to public health.

Complications The two serious complications of typhoid are liable to occur during the third week of the illness, at which time there are deep ulcers at the site of the so-called Peyer's patches in the lower part of the small intestine. The complications from these ulcers are the same as those arising from the more familiar peptic ulcers of the stomach and duodenum: an ulcer may become so deep that it **perforates** through the whole thickness of the bowel and allows faecal material to flow into the peritoneal cavity; or it may erode into a blood vessel in the wall of the bowel, causing serious **haemorrhage** into the intestine. The analogy with peptic ulcer must not be pushed too far, however, since in the third week of typhoid fever the patient is so weak and ill that perforation may occur almost silently, without causing the dramatic symptoms and signs which make the diagnosis of perforated peptic ulcer usually an easy matter. At this stage of typhoid, therefore, any sudden deterioration in the patient's general condition should draw attention to the possibility of this dangerous complication, which will almost certainly prove fatal unless the patient is operated on without delay. **Haemorrhage** is usually more easily diagnosed because of the appearance of large quantities of recognisable blood in the stools.

Treatment The prognosis of typhoid has been greatly improved since the discovery of chloramphenicol, which is usually very effective. The dose is 1.5 g twice daily by mouth for the first 5 days, then 0.75 g twice daily for a week, and finally 1 g daily for a few more days.

Nursing Care Although chloramphenicol is effective against the enteric organisms and the duration and severity of the disease have been lessened, good nursing is still of paramount importance.

The patient is strictly isolated, and every precaution must be taken to prevent the spread of infection. Disinfection of the faeces and urine and soiled linen and thorough washing of hands are the most important factors to bear in mind in this respect.

If possible the patient should be in a single room, but if in a general ward a quiet corner should be chosen conveniently near the sluice. The patient should be nursed on a sorbo mattress adequately protected with polythene. Bedclothes must be light and warm, and to prevent weight on the knees and feet a bedcradle will be necessary. The patient will rest most comfortably in a recumbent position, but if there are any signs of respiratory complications he will be propped up adequately supported by pillows.

If the toxaemia is severe the patient may be desperately ill and the most meticulous nursing care is essential. All exertion on the part of the patient must be prevented and any nursing procedure such as bathing must be carried out quickly and efficiently, so as not to tire him. The patient's position should be changed 2-hourly, to prevent pressure sores, hypostatic pneumonia and the accumulation of gas in the intestine. The danger of femoral thrombosis must also be borne in mind, and in addition to moving the patient passive movements should be given to the legs.

The tongue is coated and dry and mucus collects on the teeth. Cleaning with a solution of sodium bicarbonate and an antiseptic is necessary. All milky drinks should be followed by water and fruit drops; acid drops are particularly good, as they stimulate the flow of saliva, and so keep the mouth moist and clean.

The lips should be kept soft by applying lanoline cream. A dirty mouth may lead to such complications as suppurative parotitis or pneumonia.

During the second week, when the patient may be in the 'typhoid state', the eyes will have to be kept clean.

The temperature, pulse and respirations will be taken and recorded 4-hourly. The persistent high temperature during the second week is very exhausting, and tepid sponging will be necessary. During this treatment very careful observations are made for any signs of collapse. **Headache,** a troublesome symptom during the first week, may be relieved by shading of bright lights and application of cold compresses to the forehead. Aspirin or tab. codeine compound may be ordered. **Restlessness** may be reduced by sponging the patient with warm water, changing the position and preventing overheating by use of a bedcradle and fan. The nurse must of course remember that restlessness may be due to a full bladder, which is not appreciated by the patient in his ill state.

Bowels If constipation is present during the first week glycerine suppositories or a small enema may be ordered. During the second week diarrhoea may be severe, as the disease is reaching its height. Incontinence of urine and faeces may occur and necessitates immediate attention. The area around the anus must be frequently washed and zinc and castor oil cream must be applied as a protection. Very soft tissues or wool should be used for cleansing and absorbent pads placed under the buttocks may avoid the use of bedpans when weakness is profound. The urine should be tested daily and the output recorded. Should retention occur, catheterisation is necessary.

Diet The importance of adequate nutrition cannot be overemphasised. It is now recognised that a completely fluid diet does not prevent intestinal complications, and unless adequate nutrition is maintained the long-continued fever leads to rapid emaciation and impairs the patient's chances of recovery. The aim should be to give 2000 to 3000 calories daily and the protein content should be high. Easily digested foods, such as eggs, thin bread and butter, mashed potatoes and milk in all forms, may be given. Complan can be added to drinks and extra vitamins should be given. Minced chicken and steamed pounded fish may be introduced when the temperature is returning to normal. The nurse must vary the food as much as possible, giving small amounts frequently, and will of course feed her patient. Water and bland fluids should be given between meals; the fluid intake should be about 4 litres a day. The diet may have to be modified at various stages during the disease, according to the patient's condition. Fullness and discomfort after food, abdominal distension and tympanites or increase in the number of stools passed are indications for a more fluid diet.

Convalescence After such a debilitating illness, and because relapses do occur, the patient should be kept in bed for 10 to 14 days, and during this time leg exercises should be given. After the patient gets up the activities are gradually increased, and surprisingly soon he looks and feels extremely well.

Prevention Partial or complete immunity to the enteric fevers can be stimulated by TAB inoculations, consisting of a first intramuscular injection of 0.25 ml, followed 3 weeks later by a second injection of 0.5 ml. People who have received TAB rarely develop enteric fever, or if they do, suffer comparatively mild attacks. To be sure of continued immunity, people living in countries where the disease is endemic should have an injection of 0.5 ml of TAB every year.

Virus Infections

Chickenpox (Varicella)

The virus of chickenpox is identical or closely allied to the virus of herpes zoster (shingles); susceptible children who come into contact with shingles frequently develop chickenpox, while less frequently adult contacts of the latter disease may develop shingles.

Clinical Features After an incubation period of up to 3 weeks the rash is usually the first sign of the disease. Unlike the rash of smallpox, it is most profuse on the trunk and sparsest at the periphery of the limbs; and instead of all the lesions going through their various stages together, the spots appear in a succession of crops over several days, so that at any one time lesions can be seen at different phases of development. The spots moreover are smaller and placed more superficially in the skin than those of smallpox and they pass rapidly through the papular and vesicular stages to become pustules and then crusts within two or three days.

Clinically the disease is an extremely mild one which could not possibly be confused with classical smallpox. On the other hand, modified smallpox in a patient with partial immunity from previous vaccination may mimic it closely, and when an adult recently returned from the East develops what appears clinically to be chickenpox it is wise to seek laboratory confirmation of the diagnosis. This can be done only in laboratories specially equipped for virus work: scrapings from papules or early vesicles smeared on to clean glass slides should be sent.

Nursing Care Chickenpox is very infectious, being spread by droplet and by hands infected from the lesions.

The disease is mild, and no specific treatment is indicated; it is usually necessary to keep the patient isolated and in bed for only a few days. The irritation can be almost unbearable and is certainly the most troublesome feature. Warm boracic baths and local applications of sodium bicarbonate solution of calamine lotion may give some relief, or antihistamine tablets may be helpful.

Efforts should be made to prevent children from scratching, as the lesions quickly become infected and may then leave scars. Splinting of babies' arms may be necessary, particularly at night, and for older children cotton gloves may be useful. By day the nurse must use her ingenuity to amuse the child and take his mind off the itching.

The patient is isolated until all scabs have separated. It is not usual to isolate contacts.

Measles

Next to whooping cough this is the most serious of the infectious fevers of childhood at the present time. Passive immunity from the mother prevents infection in the first three months of life, but thereafter the child becomes highly susceptible.

Clinical Features About 10 to 14 days after exposure to infection there develops what appears to be a common cold, with fever, running nose and eyes, sneezing and cough. Examination of the mouth, however, reveals an eruption of tiny white spots like grains of salt set on a slightly reddened base, usually seen best on the mucous membrane inside the cheeks opposite the molar teeth. These are Koplik's spots, and they are diagnostic of measles. If they are overlooked the erroneous impression that the child simply has a cold may appear to be confirmed on the third day, when the temperature may come down to normal, but this opinion is finally refuted on the fourth day, when the rash appears on the skin.

The rash starts behind the ears as pink flat spots which cannot be felt with the finger (macules), about 3–5 mm in diameter, and quickly spreads over the face, trunk and limbs. Within a day or two the spots grow bigger and thicker (becoming papules), many of them coalesce into large, irregular, blotchy areas, and their colour gradually changes to a darker red. The temperature rises again with the appearance of the rash and continues for several days before finally subsiding as the spots fade. Coarse desquamation of the skin usually follows.

Complications are mainly due to secondary bacterial infection of the respiratory tract. **Broncho-pneumonia** is the most serious of them, particularly in very young children, and should always be suspected in a severely ill child with a persistent cough. **Otitis Media,** leading to a running ear, is fairly common. **Corneal ulceration** may lead to blindness, but this tragic complication can be prevented by careful treatment of any conjunctival inflammation which occurs and is very uncommon nowadays.

Treatment The virus of measles is not susceptible to any form of specific treatment, but antibiotics are of value for preventing and treating the secondary bacterial complications. It is probably wise to give a course of penicillin, starting with the appearance of the rash and continuing for up to a week. Procaine penicillin 300 000 units twice daily can be given by injection, but the oral preparation Penicillin V, 300 000 units 6-hourly is almost as satisfactory and avoids the necessity of injections.

Nursing Care Measles is highly infectious during the catarrhal stage, infection being transmitted through secretions. Paper handkerchiefs should be used and then burnt, and careful washing of hands is very important.

Nursing care aims at the prevention of complications. Strict isolation is necessary, the patient being nursed in a well-ventilated room and kept in bed for several days after the temperature has returned to normal. The room may be darkened and the bed should be placed so that the patient does not face the light because of the eye complications. Reading or anything else involving eye-strain should be strictly limited. The conjunctivae should be bathed twice daily with warm boracic lotion, after which the swabs must be burnt.

When the rash and temperature are at their height sweating may be profuse, and sponging and changing the patient will be necessary and most comforting. If there are any signs of pulmonary congestion the patient should be slightly propped up in bed; the clothing next to the skin should be non-irritating, additional warmth being given by a woollen jacket and a light blanket. To relieve irritation the skin may be sponged twice daily and then dusted with a soothing powder. The temperature, pulse and respirations will be taken 4-hourly, any increase in the respiratory rate being reported at once, since it may indicate the onset of broncho-pneumonia.

Careful observations should be made for any signs of earache or aural discharge, and the mouth and throat must be kept clean.

During the febrile stage a fluid diet is usually all the patient will want. This should be given in abundance. Once the temperature is normal it will not be long before full diet is taken.

If there are no signs of complications the patient may be allowed up in his room at the end of the first week and may mix with others a fortnight after the onset of the illness. After this disease the patient is without energy and tires very quickly, so that an adequate period of convalescence should be arranged.

Prevention *Active* immunity can be induced by giving inactivated measles vaccine 0.5 ml intramuscularly, followed one month later by 0.5 ml of live attenuated measles vaccine. These inoculations should be avoided in pregnancy and in patients with febrile illnesses. *Passive* immunity lasting about 3 weeks can be conferred by giving intramuscular gamma globulin 150–900 mg during the first 5 days after exposure to infection. Large doses prevent the attack of measles; smaller doses have the advantage that, although an attack of measles may occur, it will be a mild one and recovery from it will leave lifelong immunity.

German Measles (Rubella)

This is a less infectious disease than true measles and even in towns many people reach adult life without acquiring it. Since rubella in the first 3 months of pregnancy is often a cause of congenital defects such as deafness, cataract and heart lesions in the child, it is now recommended that girls who have not had rubella should be given a single dose of live attenuated rubella virus between the ages of 11–14. No other vaccine should be given within 3–4 weeks. This vaccine must not be given to pregnant women because of the risk of foetal damage, or to patients with Hodgkin's disease or leukaemia.

Clinical Features After an incubation period of two to three weeks the rash is usually the first indication of the disease, and takes the form of small pink macules and papules which remain distinct units and do not run together, as in true measles. There are no Koplik's spots in the mouth. The only other notable feature is generalised lymph-node enlargement, affecting particularly the nodes at the back of the neck. There are rarely any general symptoms of illness and the rash usually fades in two to three days. No **treatment** is needed.

Mumps

Mumps is a relatively trivial disease in young children, but if contracted after puberty it may have serious complications. There are undoubted advantages, therefore, in 'getting it over' early in life, and only if a child is in a weak state of health from some other illness should any steps be taken to isolate him from this infection.

Clinical Features After an incubation period of three weeks or a little longer the patient develops fever, general malaise and stiffness in the jaw, and examination reveals swelling of one or more of the salivary glands. Usually the parotid glands are affected and fill out the hollow between the angle of the jaw and the mastoid process. Sometimes the submandibular glands are affected too, or very rarely they may be involved alone. There is no rash, and usually the fever and glandular swellings subside within a few days.

Complications occur only in adolescent and adult patients and usually arise a few days after the swelling of the salivary glands. The commonest is **orchitis** (inflammation of the testicle); this is usually unilateral, but if both testicles are affected sterility may result. The comparable lesion in postpubertal girls is **oophoritis** (inflammation of the ovary) and is less common.

Mastitis (inflammation of the breast) is also occasionally seen in girls. Rare complications in either sex are **pancreatitis,** which causes severe upper abdominal pain and vomiting; and **encephalitis** (inflammation of the brain), shown by severe headache and changes in the cerebrospinal fluid, notably increase in pressure and excess of lymphocytes.

Nursing Care Infectivity is only moderate, the virus being present in the mucous secretions of nose and mouth. The infection is spread by direct contact and may be carried by crockery. There is no specific treatment.

The patient should be kept in bed as long as the temperature is raised and until the swelling subsides; this is approximately 10 days.

The mouth requires particular care, as feeding is difficult because of the pain. Fluids only can be taken, and fruit drinks may have to be avoided because they act as salivary stimulants and cause great discomfort. Milky drinks will be the main form of nourishment, and should be followed by water or a mouth wash. The mouth should be frequently rinsed with glycerine and thymol, as cleaning the mouth causes great pain. As the swelling subsides semisolid foods which do not require chewing may be given.

Warm wool or very light kaolin poultices may be applied if the swelling is painful. If there is any sign of orchitis, a scrotal support should be applied. Difficulty with micturition or retention of urine may be relieved by a warm bath. Tenderness of the breasts can be treated by applying warm wool and a supporting bandage. The patient is usually kept isolated for two weeks.

Glandular Fever

The causative agent of glandular fever has not been isolated, but it is perhaps more likely to be of viral than bacterial origin. It is quite a common disease both in children and young adults and small epidemics are frequently seen.

Clinical Features The main symptoms are fever, which is usually low and long-continued, severe lassitude, general malaise and sometimes sore throat. Examination reveals enlarged lymph-nodes in the neck and elsewhere and the spleen can often be felt. The white blood count shows an excess of lymphocytes, among which some abnormal 'glandular fever cells' can usually be seen and are a very important diagnostic finding. The **Paul-Bunnell** test is usually positive: the patient's serum even in a titre (or dilution) of 1 : 64 or more causes clumping and haemolysis of sheep's red cells.

Treatment There is no specific treatment. Complete recovery always occurs, though frequently the patient continues to feel rather weak and tired for several months.

Dysentery

Bacillary Dysentery

This is an acute infection of the colon which is spread by infected food or water. Like enteric fever it is common therefore in countries with poor sanitation, and throughout history epidemics have afflicted armies in the field. In this country it is rarely seen except in institutions, such as mental hospitals.

There are three types of dysentery bacillus: **Shiga** causes the most severe infection; **Flexner** dysentery is usually less serious, though fatal cases are not unknown; **Sonne** is the mildest variety and is the one found in Britain.

Clinical Features The incubation period is up to 1 week. The disease starts abruptly, and in its severest form causes high fever, vomiting, profuse diarrhoea with blood and mucus in the stools, dehydration and sometimes collapse and death within a few hours. At the other end of the scale Sonne dysentery as seen in this country causes slight fever, diarrhoea and vomiting with attacks of colicky abdominal pain, but without any serious constitutional symptoms, and recovery invariably occurs within a week or so. **Diagnosis** is confirmed by isolation of the specific organism from culture of the stools.

Treatment Mild dysentery is best treated symptomatically since there is no evidence that antibiotics speed recovery. Antibiotics are given to patients with severe infections, but as resistant strains are common the organism must first be isolated so that its sensitivity to antibiotics may be tested. The drugs used include tetracycline 500 mg 6-hourly, oral streptomycin 0.5 g 6-hourly and ampicillin 500 mg 6-hourly.

Nursing Care The patient is nursed in a bed conveniently near the sanitary block. The patient may or may not be extremely ill, but in either case the most conscientious nursing care is essential to prevent the spread of infection. Disinfection of excreta and soiled linen and scrupulous care in washing hands are the important measures, and facilities must be provided for the patient to wash his hands immediately after using a bedpan.

Bowels The number and nature of the stools must be noted. A bedpan should be available at the shortest notice; and if stools are so frequent that the patient becomes too exhausted to be constantly using a bedpan, absorbent pads of wool and tissue should be placed under the buttocks and changed frequently.

Excoriation of the skin round the anus must be prevented by washing carefully or cleaning with olive oil, followed by application of a protective cream such as zinc and castor oil.

Kaolin, kaolin and morphia mixture and codeine phosphate are all useful in controlling diarrhoea, and in severe cases tinct. opii may be ordered.

Diet Fluid diet only should be given at first, and indeed the patient will have no appetite for solids. He will have to be persuaded to drink sufficient fluid to balance fluid loss, and therefore the amount taken must be recorded. All drinks must be cool to avoid stimulating the activity of the intestine. As the symptoms subside, semisolid non-residue foods with a high protein content may be given. Gradually it may be increased to a normal diet, though high residue foods should be avoided for a week or two.

Once the diarrhoea stops, the patient quickly improves. If in a single room he may be allowed up, but isolation is still necessary until three consecutive negative stools have been obtained over a period of a few days.

Amoebic Dysentery

Unlike bacillary dysentery, this is a chronic disease which is extremely difficult to eradicate completely, and although it occurs mainly in the tropics, it is seen not infrequently in this country in patients who have at one time lived in the East.

It is due to a protozoon, *Entamoeba histolytica*, which exists in two forms: the active (or vegetative) form lives in the ulcers in the colon and can be found in the mucous exudate in the faeces, though it dies as soon as the stool becomes cool; the resting (or cystic) form survives for weeks or months after being passed in the faeces and by contaminating food or water is responsible for transmitting the disease to other people.

Clinical Features Mild but persistent looseness of the stools, with vague colicky lower abdominal pains and general lassitude, are the usual symptoms, which over a period of months or years show considerable fluctuations in severity. Sometimes an exacerbation of abdominal pain associated with tenderness over the caecum may make the diagnosis from acute appendicitis extremely difficult.

Diagnosis The best way of confirming the diagnosis is by demonstrating active vegetative *Entamoeba histolytica* (EH) in the stools. This is done by examining under the microscope a little mucus from a fresh faecal specimen; and as there will be no hope of finding active EH if the stool has had time to cool, the patient must be sent to defaecate in the laboratory so that the examination can be carried out with the minimum of delay. Alternatively, a specimen of mucus for examination may be obtained by **sigmoidoscopy,** and whenever this investigation is done on a patient with suspected amoebiasis a microscope should be at hand for immediate use if necessary. In addition the finding of antibodies to *Entamoeba histolytica* in the blood is useful confirmatory evidence of infection.

Complications The most important complication is amoebic hepatitis, which may proceed to the formation of an amoebic abscess in the liver. This is often an extremely difficult condition to recognise, since the underlying disease in the colon may have caused only trivial symptoms; and although some patients do have fever with striking pain and tenderness over the liver, in other cases the disease may remain clinically silent until quite an advanced stage has been reached.

Treatment Metronidazole is a safe and effective amoebicide which has replaced emetine as the drug of first choice in this disease. It is given by mouth in doses of 400–800 mg t.d.s. for 10 days. Older regimes of treatment such as the following are still occasionally used:

Days 1–3:	Emetine hydrochloride (EBI) 60 mg IM daily.
Days 1–5:	Tetracycline 250 mg 6-hourly.
Days 6–16:	Emetine bismuth iodide 200 mg daily by mouth.
Days 14–35:	Diodoquin tabs. 600 mg t.d.s

Emetine by injection may have toxic effects on the myocardium and the patient should be kept in bed while it is being given. To minimise the vomiting caused by EBI the drug is given at bedtime with an antihistamine such as promethazine 25 mg and a sedative such as amylobarbitone 200 mg.

13

Caring for Mentally Ill Patients

by D. STAFFORD-CLARK, MD, FRCP, DPM

It is not the purpose of this book to describe the phenomena of mental illness in any detail, or to enter into descriptions of psychiatric treatment. An appropriate textbook must be consulted for adequate accounts of mental illness and psychiatric nursing, but the following observations may help the nurse in general training, who will have to rely essentially upon tact, patience, compassion and a sympathetic and imaginative understanding when dealing with patients who are mentally ill.

Such illness can be regarded as including the whole range of disturbance of human emotion, judgement, action and personality, whenever this disturbance is sufficiently profound to be considered abnormal. As encountered by the nurse in general training, it will probably present itself either as a relatively acute disturbance of normal contact with reality, secondary to the toxic effects upon the brain of intercurrent physical disease (being then called delirium, or a toxic confusional state); or as an exaggerated emotional response to the stresses of pain, fear or personal unhappiness.

The former type of reaction is an example of what is often described as a **psychosis;** that is, a form of mental illness, whether acute or chronic, which actually interferes with the patient's understanding and appreciation of what is going on in the world about him. By contrast, disorders of the latter kind, wherein patients are abnormally emotionally vulnerable or upset but do not lose touch with external reality, are called **neuroses.**

Both kinds of patients require, above all, kindness and acceptance of their symptoms without alarm or hostility. To achieve this, it is necessary to understand something of the nature of the symptoms themselves. Among the more important are: confusion, with clouding of consciousness, and disorientation in space or time; excitement or stupor; delusions, hallucinations and illusions; depression or elation of mood; disorders of thinking; and disturbed or impulsive conduct.

Confusion, with Clouding of Consciousness, and Disorientation in Space or Time

These symptoms are most commonly seen in patients whose brain function is disturbed by toxic changes or physical damage. They are therefore prominent in states of delirium, in which patients may become progressively restless, alarmed and alarming, as they lose touch with their situation, not knowing where they are, why they are there or how long they have been there. The intensity of the symptoms tends to increase with the approach of night, and sustained personal contact, adequate light without shadows and reassuring tolerance of their restlessness and noisiness usually make nursing in a single room or side-ward essential. Acute conditions of this kind, adequately treated, usually subside within two or three days.

Excitement or stupor are both essentially disturbances of conduct. In both cases there is a corresponding underlying disturbance of mind; but often the patient is inaccessible to discussion, or even emotional contact with others, and we can only then proceed upon the basis of treating the condition as the patient's behaviour demands, bearing in mind that anything we do must be justified by being required for the safety, well-being and ultimate recovery of the patient himself, or for the safety and well-being of others. Following recovery from such states of excitement or stupor, a patient previously inaccessible may often say that despite his inability at that time to communicate with others, or to modify his conduct, he was aware of what was going on, and may have been helped by the calmness and confident acceptance of his needs by those who looked after him during his critical illness.

Delusions, hallucinations and illusions may well occur as symptoms of psychotic illness, whether acute or chronic. A delusion may be defined as a false or mistaken belief, which has for the patient the force of conviction, and is firmly held despite all evidence to the contrary. A hallucination is a perception through one of the senses, which does not correspond to any stimulus in the outside world; whereas an illusion is a similar perception, which, although produced by an external stimulus, is misinterpreted by the patient in purely subjective terms.

Examples will make these three descriptive terms clear. If a man believes that he has lost all his money, is being kept under constant observation by unknown enemies through radar or television and is having his food poisoned, or the air in his room contaminated by gas pumped through the ceiling, and if he cannot be induced to modify these beliefs, although they remain demonstrably untrue, then he is suffering from delusions. If he hears voices or sees visions, which no one else can hear or see, or smells, for example, the gas which he believes to be entering his room, and if these experiences are in fact projections of his own fantasy, released by illness, then he is hallucinated. If, on the other hand, he mistakes his doctor or nurse for his father or mother, or for the devil come to take him away, then he is suffering from illusions, which are being grafted on to the normal experience of seeing people, whose identity he misconstrues.

Depression of mood is obviously not exclusive to mental illness, occurring in many cases in response to the patient's life situation. However, it may appear without such apparent external justification, or it may persist after some external catastrophe, such as bereavement or personal loss or disaster, to a point where the patient is clearly no longer reacting in a normal way. If such depression cannot be recognised by the patient as without justification, and furthermore cannot be lastingly relieved by any form of comfort or reasonable reassurance, it strongly suggests mental illness. When encountered as a symptom of such illness it needs, *not exhortations to the patient to be sensible or to pull himself together*, but rather an acceptance of this symptom as a form of mental pain, for which comfort and reassurance are appropriate, but for which exhortation or criticism *are entirely out of place* and in fact likely to be thoroughly harmful. *It has to be remembered that depression, which involves a divorce of the patient's judgement from reality, is perhaps the single most important cause of a state of sufficient suffering and hopelessness to lead to suicide.*

Exaltation or pathological elation, which has to be distinguished from sheer excitement, represents the opposite kind of disorder of mood. Once again, when justified by the circumstances, and normally short-lived, it is clearly separable from mental imbalance of any kind. But if not related to the reality of the patient's personal situation, it will again often be seen to overthrow judgement and to lead to conduct characteristic of mental illness.

Disorders of thinking occur when the patient's capacity to maintain a train of thought is constantly interrupted; a symptom of mental illness which differs only in intensity from the normal preoccupations and difficulty in thinking which we are all apt to experience when we are fatigued. Other forms of disorder of thought include those in which the patient relates every external circumstance to himself, and believes that everything that happens has some special meaning directed towards him. This kind of thought disorder leads naturally to delusions, in explanation of the otherwise incomprehensible picture of the world which the patient receives.

Bizarre and impulsive conduct may be the outcome of delusions and hallucinations, and often represents the patient's single-handed attempt to cope with a world which has become unbearable, terrifying, threatening and beyond control.

All these considerations should enable us to approach the patient with mental illness with more confidence, more compassion and, above all, more understanding than would come naturally to an individual who took normal contact with reality for granted, and was unable or unwilling to believe that illness could disturb it. The art of nursing the mentally ill patient is really the art of accepting the isolation, the distortion of reality and often the loneliness, fear and need for acceptance and confidence on the part of other people, which are so characteristic of the patient troubled with mental illness.

It is very rare indeed for such patients to be dangerous to others, despite the popular belief. Even when, because of their delusions or hallucinations, they may feel threatened, and therefore may equally feel bound to defend themselves, calmness, kindness, confidence and understanding will nearly always bridge the gulf, and enable someone who can exert and display these qualities to deal successfully with even the most disturbed patient.

14
Venereal Diseases

The word venereal is derived from Venus, the goddess of love, and is applied to those diseases which are communicated by sexual intercourse. The important members of this group are gonorrhoea, syphilis and non-specific urethritis; others much rarer in this country are soft sore and lymphogranuloma inguinale.

Gonorrhoea

The *Neisseria gonorrhoeae* is a delicate organism which does not survive for long outside the body, and gonorrhoea in the adult is almost invariably the result of coitus with an infected person. Recovery confers no immunity and it is therefore possible for the same person to have repeated attacks of the disease. Young girls may acquire the disease from infected bed linen, but outbreaks of vulvo-vaginitis in children are in fact more often due to other organisms.

Clinical Features (1) **In Men.** Within about 3–10 days of exposure to infection the first symptom is usually slight scalding on micturition, soon followed by a purulent urethral discharge and the appearance of tender swollen lymph-nodes in the groins. If specific treatment is not given the infection may extend back to the posterior part of the urethra and prostate gland, leading to chronic prostatitis and eventually in some cases to urethral stricture. Complications in other parts of the body include acute arthritis, usually affecting one of the large joints of the limbs, and iritis.

(2) **In Women,** after a similar incubation period, the disease usually presents with painful frequent micturition and vaginal discharge, though there may be no symptoms if the infection is confined to the cervix. If untreated the infection may spread into the uterus and Fallopian tubes; an acute abscess may form in one of the tubes, known as a pyosalpinx, and subsequent sealing of the tubes by fibrosis may cause sterility.

Diagnosis is confirmed by bacteriological identification of gonococci in smears of pus from the lesions.

Treatment Acute gonorrhoea is cured by 1 day's treatment with penicillin, a single injection of procaine penicillin 1.2–2.4 g (1 200 000–2 400 000 units) being usually sufficient. It is important to remember that this treatment may suppress the appearance of a syphilitic infection acquired at the same time; and as it will be quite inadequate for the cure of syphilis, serological tests for the latter disease must always be made 3 and 6 months after the gonorrhoea has been treated.

Gonorrhoeal ophthalmia neonatorum is prevented by the instillation of penicillin drops into the eyes of newborn babies.

Syphilis

As a result of improved methods of treatment and the consequent reduced infectivity of patients with the disease, syphilis is now quite rare. It remains very important, however, because of the serious lesions which may appear in almost any organ of the body many years after the primary infection.

The organism is a spirochaete (*Treponema pallidum*), and is transmitted only by direct contact. **Congenital syphilis** is contracted by the foetus through the placenta in the later months of pregnancy; **acquired syphilis** is nearly always the result of sexual intercourse with an infected person, though occasionally extragenital infection may be acquired, for example by doctors or nurses, from handling syphilitic lesions.

Congenital Syphilis

Fortunately this disease is extremely rare nowadays. It is preventible, since if a woman with syphilis is given adequate treatment sufficiently early in pregnancy, the child will escape infection. Routine serological tests should therefore be done on all women on their first attendance at an antenatal clinic.

Clinical Features The syphilitic infant fails to gain weight normally in the first month or two and may have an infection of the nose (known as 'snuffles'), which retards the development of the nasal bones and leads eventually to a depressed bridge of the nose, which is a permanent and highly characteristic stigma of the disease. A scaly yellow or copper-coloured rash is also common. Among the many lesions which may appear later in childhood are notches in the incisor teeth of the second dentition (Hutchinson's teeth), scars known as rhagades radiating from the margins of the lips, and interstitial keratitis (inflammation of the cornea of the eye, often referred to as 'IK').

Acquired Syphilis

Acquired syphilis passes through three stages, known as **primary** syphilis, **secondary** syphilis and **tertiary** syphilis. The secondary stage is seen a month or two after the primary lesion, but many years may elapse before a tertiary lesion appears.

Primary syphilis is characterised by the appearance of a hard sore known as a chancre (pronounced 'shanker') about a month after exposure to infection. In men the chancre usually occurs on the penis; in women it appears most often on the labia or cervix, and in the latter situation readily escapes notice. Much more rarely the primary sore may be on the lip, tongue or nipple. The chancre is a hard, painless ulcer about 1 cm in diameter, has a thin, serous discharge and is accompanied by painless enlargement of the regional lymph-nodes.

The diagnosis is established by demonstrating spirochaetes in the serous discharge from the chancre by a microscopic technique known as dark-ground illumination (DGI).

Secondary syphilis may cause some constitutional disturbance with sore throat, low fever and generalised lymph-node enlargement, but usually its manifestations are confined to the skin and the mucous membrane of the mouth. Various types of skin rash are seen, all having in common a symmetrical distribution over the body, absence of irritation and a colour usually likened to raw ham. In the mouth painless, slimy, greyish patches known as 'snail-track ulcers' are the typical lesions. Warty lesions known as condylomata may appear in the peri-anal and vulval regions. The lesions on the skin and mucosal ulcers in the secondary stage are highly infective and serological tests for syphilis are invariably positive.

Tertiary syphilis A localised swelling known as a **gumma** may appear anywhere in the body many years after the primary infection; these lesions differ from those of primary and secondary syphilis in containing no spirochaetes and being therefore non-infective. In certain situations, such as the liver, the lung or the stomach, a gumma may be mistaken for a carcinoma; the distinction can be made by giving potassium iodide 2–4 g daily, which causes rapid disappearance of a gumma but has no effect on a carcinoma. The centre of a gumma often breaks down and leads to the formation of an ulcer with sharply punched out margins.

Syphilitic aortitis is discussed on p. 24 and neurosyphilis on p. 155.

Treatment of Syphilis

The standard treatment for syphilis at the present time is an intensive course of penicillin, consisting of 500 000–1 000 000 units daily for 8–10 days. It is extremely important to repeat the Wassermann reaction in the blood every 3–6 months for the next 2 years, and on at least one occasion during that period to examine the CSF. If any positive results are obtained from these tests a further course of penicillin is indicated.

Non-specific Urethritis

Following the striking decline in numbers of patients with gonorrhoea and syphilis, non-specific urethritis is now one of the commonest conditions seen in VD departments. Comparatively little is known about this disease, but it is probably of virus origin and is certainly acquired by sexual intercourse. It is seen mainly in young men.

After a variable incubation period, which can probably be as long as 2–3 months, the patient develops scalding, frequency and a urethral discharge which contains no gonococci or other specific organisms. In addition to urethral discharge some patients have conjunctivitis and acute arthritis affecting one of the large joints of the limbs, and the condition is then known as **Reiter's syndrome.**

Treatment There is no specific treatment. The urethral discharge usually subsides fairly quickly, but the arthritis when present may persist for many months.

Genital Herpes

Genital herpes is due to herpes simplex virus (HSV1 or HSV2) which has the ability to remain latent in the tissues so that, as with cold sores, relapses are common. The infection is acquired by sexual intercourse and has recently become much more common, possibly because of the more widespread practice of orogenital contact.

Primary infection may be heralded by a flu-like illness with fever, malaise and aching followed by the appearance on the genitalia of papules which become vesicular in a few days and then rupture forming painful ulcers. In women they may cause such painful dysuria as to inhibit micturition.

Relapses occur in about half the patients and may be precipitated by fever, exposure to UVL, trauma, menstruation or stress. They are usually less severe than the first attack.

Carcinoma of the Cervix It has been suggested, but not proved, that HSV infection is a factor in the development of cervical cancer and women with genital herpes are advised to have annual cervical smears examined.

Treatment An analgesic jelly (Lidothesin gel) may be very helpful in women with difficulty in micturition due to pain. Specific treatment with acyclovir relieves symptoms and promotes healing but does not prevent relapses.

Soft Sore (Chancroid)

This is very rare in Britain, though it is occasionally seen in seaports. The important thing is to distinguish it from the hard sore or chancre of syphilis: this is done bacteriologically, since the specific organism (Ducrey's bacillus) can be isolated from soft sore, whereas serum from it contains no spirochaetes on dark-ground illumination. The lesion usually responds satisfactorily to a course of sulphadimidine by mouth.

Lymphogranuloma Inguinale

This is also very rare in Britain. It is a virus infection with an incubation period of up to two weeks. The initial lesion is a small vesicle usually on the penis, followed two or three weeks later by enlargement of the lymph-nodes in the groin. This swelling may become quite massive and eventually suppuration may occur with the discharge of yellow pus through multiple sinuses on the skin. There is often quite severe constitutional reaction with high fever. In women inflammation of the rectum (proctitis) and subsequent rectal stricture may occur.

The Frei skin test is positive in nearly all cases.

Treatment Most patients respond satisfactorily to a course of oral sulphadimidine, aureomycin or terramycin, but occasionally surgical incision and curetting of the suppurating lymph-nodes become necessary.

Social and Nursing Aspects of Venereal Disease

Venereal disease is not notifiable in this country nor is the treatment of contacts any longer compulsory. It is of particular importance to persuade those who are infected to come for treatment and those who are possible contacts to come for investigation. In large cities lists of clinics are easily available and treatment is free and confidential. It is preferable for the patient if the special clinic is attached to a general hospital, as this makes it easier for him to ask for time off work without disclosing where he is going; ideally, of course, the clinic should be (and normally is) at such an hour that he can attend it after work.

Dealing with the patient in the clinic calls for great tact and kindness. Many patients feel bitterly ashamed of having contracted the disease, others are equally emotionally upset but express their feelings in apparent bravado and defiance. A slightly matter-of-fact but firm attitude is often more successful than an over-sentimental one. It is not the province of the nurse to pass moral judgements on her patients, and the way in which the patient became infected is of less immediate concern than persuading the patient to complete her treatment. It is difficult not to become exasperated with the patient who is constantly reinfected, and the nurse must realise that she is very rarely able to alter her patient's easy-going attitude to life. Because of this irresponsible attitude, a vital part of the work of the clinic is tracing contacts and following up patients who default during treatment. Many patients do not realise that although their symptoms are relieved they may still be infectious.

Tracing these people is normally the work of a health visitor or specially trained medical social worker; these may be combined with other duties or in a large area will be full-time work. The greatest tact is necessary when doing this work as the object of the visit must never be disclosed to anyone but the patient.

In the clinic, apart from receiving specific treatment the patient should be given advice about preventing the spread of infection; for example, in gonorrhoea simple measures, such as the use of a separate towel and wash-cloth, the wearing of pads which must be carefully disposed of and washing the hands if they have become contaminated, should all be carefully explained to the patient. The special risk to any little girls in the household, particularly if they share an adult's bed, should be pointed out. If the living conditions are bad or unsuitable (for example, if the patient is living in a lodging house), the patient may even have to be admitted to hospital for a few days. The same precautions apply in the second stage of syphilis, and in addition the patient with lesions in the mucous membrane of the mouth should use separate crockery and tooth-mug until his mouth is no longer infectious. If it proves necessary for any reason to admit the patient, nurses should remember that barrier precautions are designed to prevent the spread of infection from the place where the lesions are. In one case the appropriate measure may be the provision of a separate bedpan, in another of separate crockery, cutlery and toilet articles.

Publicity about venereal disease presents another problem. Many adults have no idea what venereal disease is, quite apart from knowing how it is spread; wider dissemination of the true facts among the public would bring many people to realise the dangers of promiscuous intercourse and the importance of early treatment, not only for the sake of their own health, but to prevent the infection of other people.

15

Diseases Due to Worms (HELMINTHS)

Tapeworms (Cestodes)

In order to complete their life-cycle these parasites have to inhabit the bodies of two separate and unwilling 'hosts'. The adult tapeworm lives in the intestine of the main host, its ova passing out with the faeces. If these ova are ingested by a suitable 'intermediate host', the larval forms of the worm hatch out, gain access to the bloodstream and are distributed throughout the muscles of the body. Now if the intermediate host is eaten by a 'main host' the cysts in its muscles develop into adult tapeworms in the intestine of the latter.

Man acts as the main host for three tapeworms, *Taenia saginata*, the common beef tapeworm, *Taenia solium*, the less common pork tapeworm and *Diphyllobothrium latum*, the fish tapeworm.

T. saginata and T. solium

These are the only tapeworms likely to be found in this country and infection is acquired by eating respectively imperfectly cooked beef or pork containing the larval forms. These tapeworms are white, flat, ribbon-like structures, about 1 cm wide and many yards long, subdivided into a large number of segments some of which break off from time to time and appear in the faeces. The head, which is no more than a pin-head in size, is firmly attached to the duodenum or upper part of the jejunum.

Clinical Features There may be some abdominal discomfort or diarrhoea, but frequently the patient has no symptoms until he notices segments of the worm in his stools. A white cell blood count sometimes shows an increase in the eosinophil cells.

Diagnosis is established by the identification of segments or ova of the tapeworm in the faeces.

Treatment (*a*) *T. solium.* After being kept on a fluid diet for two days the patient is given extract of filix mas. The dose for an adult is 8 ml diluted in a suitably flavoured draught. He is then given a strong dose of salts. The stools should be strained through black muslin and a search made for the head of the worm, for if this has not been dislodged the worm will grow again to its previous length in two to three months.

(*b*) *T. saginata.* Two tablets of niclosamide (0.5 g each) are chewed and swallowed, followed by two more in an hour. No preliminary starvation is needed.

Cysticercosis is the disease which results when man acts as the intermediate host for *T. solium.* The cysts of the larval forms are found throughout the muscles of the body, and in the brain; in the latter situation they may be a cause of epileptic fits. In this country cysticercosis is seen in soldiers who have served for many years in India.

Hydatid Disease

Here man is acting as the intermediate host for a minute tapeworm whose adult form (*Taenia echinococcus*) lives in the intestine of dogs and other carnivorous animals. It causes large cysts in the lung, liver, brain or, more rarely, in other organs.

Round Worms (Nematodes)

Round worms are so called because they are round in cross section instead of being flat like the tapeworms. There are many different types, but the commonest is:

Ascaris lumbricoides

This worm is about 15–25 cm long. It lives in the intestine and its ova can be found in the faeces. There is no intermediate host, its life-cycle being completed if ova are transmitted to the mouth of the human host as a result of faecal contamination of the fingers.

Treatment A single dose of piperazine is effective, 3.0 g for a young child or 4.0 g for an older child or adult. The drug acts by paralysing the muscle of the worm, which is passed alive per rectum.

Trichinosis

The adult form of this minute round worm (*Trichinella spiralis*) lives in the intestine of the pig; embryo worms find their way into the animal's blood stream and develop into small cysts, about ½ mm long, in the muscles. If inadequately cooked pork from such a pig is eaten, an adult worm develops in the human intestine, and in time its embryos are disseminated in the bloodstream throughout the body.

Clinical Features Small localised outbreaks occur from the eating of pork from an infected animal; pork sausage-meat, either fried too hastily or actually eaten raw, has a bad reputation in this connection. About a week later (when the embryos are passing into the muscles) there is fever, muscular pain and tenderness and frequently oedema of the eyelids and 'splinter haemorrhages' under the nails. The blood always shows a great excess of eosinophil cells.

Diagnosis can sometimes be established by identification of the encysted larvae in a piece of muscle removed for biopsy.

Treatment is purely symptomatic.

Toxocariasis

The adult stage of the worms *Toxocara canis* and *Toxocara cati* live in the intestines of dogs and cats respectively. Ova pass out in the animal's faeces and human infestation occurs from soil-contaminated fingers or food. The ova develop in the human intestine into larvae which penetrate the mucosa and may be carried to any organ in the body. Children are particularly at risk from sucking contaminated fingers. The organ most often damaged is the eye: permanent impairment or loss of vision may result from choroidoretinitis.

The **diagnosis** is supported by the finding of eosinophilia and Toxocaral antibodies in the blood.

Treatment Diethylcarbamazine 3 mg/kg body weight given three times daily for 21 days will kill the larvae, but cannot of course undo damage to vital structures such as the eye.

Glossary

Acyanotic. Having no cyanosis.

Agranulocytosis. Absence from the blood of the granulocyte (or polymorph) leucocytes.

Allergy. A state of abnormal sensitivity to some substance, contact with which causes various symptoms and signs.

Anaphylactic shock. A severe reaction occurring in an allergic subject after injection of serum or other foreign proteins.

Anuria. Failure of the kidneys to secrete any urine.

Aphasia. Inability to speak.

Arrhythmia. Irregularity of rhythm.

Bronchogram. A chest X-ray taken after filling the bronchi with a fluid which renders them visible on the X-ray plate.

Bronchoscopy. Examination of the trachea and bronchi through an instrument (a bronchoscope) passed through the mouth.

Bullae. Blisters in the epidermis which contain watery fluid and are more than about half a centimetre in diameter.

Cardiac Output. The amount of blood discharged in a unit of time by each of the ventricles of the heart.

Colic. Spasmodic pain due to excessive muscular contractions in either the intestines, the bile ducts, the ureters or the uterus.

Diastole. The interval between two contractions (systoles) of the heart.

Diuresis. Increased production of urine by the kidneys. Hence **Diuretic:** a drug which increases the urinary output.

Dysarthria. Slurring of speech.

Dysphagia. Difficulty in swallowing.

Electrocardiograph. A tracing of the electrical changes associated with the beating of the heart.

Embolus. A piece of blood-clot or other foreign body circulating in the blood. Hence **Embolism:** the plugging of an artery by an embolus.

Emphysema. A state of over-distension and loss of elasticity of the lungs.

Exophthalmos (or **Proptosis**). Forward protrusion of the eyeball.

Gastroscopy. Examination of the gastric mucous membrane through an instrument (a gastroscope) passed through the mouth and oesophagus into the stomach.

Haematemesis. Vomiting of blood.

Haemoptysis. Coughing up of blood.

Hormone. A substance secreted into the blood which has some special effect on another part of the body.

Hyperchromic. Having excess of colour (applied to red cells which contain more haemoglobin than normal).

Hyperglycaemia. An excess of sugar in the blood.

Hyperplasia. An overgrowth of tissue resulting from an increase in the number of its cells.

Hypertrophy. An overgrowth of tissue resulting from an increase in the size of its cells.

Hypochromic. Having too little colour (applied to red cells which contain less haemoglobin than normal).

Hypoglycaemia. An abnormally low level of sugar in the blood.

Idiosyncrasy. An abnormal or excessive reaction to a drug.

Infarct. A piece of tissue which has died from lack of oxygen after its arterial blood supply has been cut off by thrombosis or embolism. Hence **Infarction:** the formation of an infarct.

Leucocytosis. An excessive number of white cells in the blood.

Leucopenia. Abnormally few white cells in the blood.

Macrocytic. Having large cells.

Macules. Spots which are not raised above the level of the surrounding skin.

Microcytic. Having small cells.

Oliguria. Diminished secretion of urine by the kidneys.

Osmosis. The diffusion of fluids through a semipermeable membrane. Hence **Osmotic pressure:** the pressure exerted by certain substances which cannot pass through the membrane to draw through the membrane a certain volume of fluid from the other side (e.g. the effect of plasma proteins in 'pulling' tissue fluid into the blood).

Papules. 'Solid' spots which are raised above the level of the surrounding skin.

Proctoscopy. Examination of the rectum through an instrument (a proctoscope) introduced through the anus.

Purpura. A bleeding disease showing haemorrhage into the skin.

Pustules. Small localised collections of pus in the epidermis.

Pyogenic. Causing the formation of pus.

Refractory period. A short interval after each beat of the heart in which the heart-muscle will not respond to any other stimulus.

Sigmoidoscopy. Similar to protoscopy but performed with a much longer instrument (a sigmoidoscope) which enables the bowel to be examined up to 30 cm (12 inches) from the anus.

Status asthmaticus. A severe attack of asthma which has persisted for more than 24 hours and has not responded to the usual antispasmodic remedies.

Status epilepticus. A succession of epileptic convulsions without recovery of consciousness between them.

Syndrome. A group of symptoms and signs forming a typical clinical picture.

Systole. The phase of contraction of the heart.

Tetanus. An infection occurring mainly in deep puncture wounds contaminated with soil and characterised by widespread muscular spasm and convulsions.

Tetany. A state of abnormal muscular irritability due to a deficiency of calcium in the blood and characterised by painful cramps in the hands and feet (carpopedal spasms). In **Latent tetany** the patient has no spontaneous symptoms, but the muscular irritability can be demonstrated by special tests.

Thrombocytopenia. Deficiency of blood platelets (or thrombocytes).

Thrombosis. The clotting of blood in a blood vessel. Hence **Thrombus:** a blood-clot.

Vesicles. Small blisters in the epidermis which contain watery fluid and are less than half a centimetre in diameter.

Diets

High Fibre Diet

Instructions for Using Bran

1 One heaped teaspoon bran 3 times a day before meals or with the first course.
2 Increase the dose after 1 week by one heaped teaspoon bran.
3 Continue to increase the dose by one heaped teaspoon each week until the motions are of a soft consistency and passed without effort.

You may experience some flatulence or wind at first, but this will pass. DO NOT STOP TAKING THE BRAN ON THIS ACCOUNT.

The amount of bran necessary depends on the quantity of fibre in the rest of your diet. Once you have found the correct dose of bran for yourself continue to take this indefinitely unless directed otherwise by your doctor.

Some Ways of Taking Bran

1 Dry, but washed down with a glass of water, milk, fruit juice or other liquid.
2 Moisten bran with a small amount of boiling water and then add to food/drink.
3 Mixed with breakfast cereal.
4 In soup, e.g. mixed vegetable soup, lentil soup, scotch broth.
5 In home-made bread, cakes and biscuits—approximately 1½ oz (45 g) bran should be added to each 1 lb (460 g) 100% extraction wholemeal flour.
6 In sauces, milk puddings and stewed fruit. (The bran may alter the appearance.)

Foods with a High Fibre Content

Breakfast Cereals	Porridge oats, Weetabix, Shredded Wheat, All Bran, muesli.
Flour	Wholewheat or whole rye (100% extraction), e.g. Allinsons, Prewett's.

Bread	Any made from wholewheat or whole rye flour (100% extraction). Most so-called wholemeal bread is not made of whole grain flour.
Rice	Use brown rice if you can. Otherwise, add bran to white rice.
Cakes and Biscuits	Use wholewheat flour, oatmeal or rolled oats with dried fruit and nuts. Digestive biscuits, whole-grain crispbread, e.g. Ryvita.
Fruits	All kinds—in generous amounts and raw, with the skins where possible; also dried fruit.
Vegetables	All kinds—in generous amounts. As much raw as possible. Potatoes should be baked in their skins or boiled in their skins.
Pulses	Peas, lentils, beans, e.g. Butter, Red Kidney, Haricot, Black Eye, Aduki, Crab Eye, Mung and Soya Beans.
Soups	Those made with vegetables, preferably home-made.
Nuts	All kinds.

Suggested Meal Pattern

Breakfast	Porridge or high fibre cereal Serving of egg, bacon, ham or fish Tomatoes or mushrooms, if desired Bread made with 100% wholewheat flour, toasted, if desired Butter or margarine Coarse marmalade Tea or coffee or fruit juice
Mid-morning	Tea or coffee or milk or fruit juice Digestive biscuits, if desired, or fresh fruit
Lunch/ Evening Meal	Serving of home-made vegetable soup Serving of meat or chicken or fish or egg or cheese Serving of potatoes cooked in their skins (eat the skin) Large helping of. lightly cooked vegetables or salad *or* Snack lunch e.g. salad, sandwiches or snack on toast—all with wholemeal bread

	Fresh or stewed fruit or pudding made with fruit or nuts Tea or coffee or fruit juice
Tea	Tea with milk Wholewheat bread or crispbread e.g. Ryvita Butter or margarine Home-made cake or biscuit made with wholewheat flour, if desired
Bedtime	Tea, coffee or bedtime drink Digestive biscuits or fresh fruit, if desired

Ensure that an adequate fluid intake is taken daily—at least *8 cups*, in the form of tea, coffee, water, fruit juice, etc.

Low Sodium Diet (500 mg)

Breakfast

Raw or stewed fruit or tomatoes if desired.
Unsalted oatmeal or Shredded Wheat with milk from daily allowance.
1 egg or a portion of unsalted fish.
Salt-free bread and butter. Jam or marmalade.
Tea or coffee.

Mid-morning

Tea, coffee or fruit.
Salt-free bread and butter, if desired.

Lunch

Average helping of meat or fish.
Any fresh vegetable cooked without salt.
Raw or stewed fruit or water jelly.
Tea or coffee, if desired.

Tea

Salt-free bread and butter or Motza biscuits.
Jam or salad.
Tea.

Supper

Average helping of meat, fish, egg or unsalted cream cheese.
Unsalted fresh vegetables or salad.
Salt-free bread and butter, if desired.
Raw or stewed fruit or water jelly.
Tea if desired.

Daily

Milk, not more than 300 ml.

Note:—If ordinary bread is used instead of salt-free bread the sodium content of this diet is 800–1000 mg.

Foods allowed without restriction

Fruit, sugar, jam, marmalade, honey, boiled sweets, barley sugar.
Salt-free bread, Energen rolls, Motza biscuits.
Salt-free butter, vegetarian or Kosher margarine.
Unsalted vegetables, fresh or frozen.
Unsalted boiled rice, macaroni or spaghetti.

Foods to Avoid

Salt in cooking or on plate.
Ordinary bread and biscuits, including Ryvita and Vita-Wheat.
All prepared breakfast cereals, except Shredded Wheat, Puffed Wheat or Puffed Rice.
Puddings, cakes and scones made with baking powder.
Tinned meat or fish, shellfish, smoked haddock, kippers, bloaters.
Cheese (unless unsalted), bacon, ham, sausages, meat or fish pastes.
Tinned vegetables.
Bovril, Oxo, Marmite, gravy powders, salad dressing, pickles and sauces.
Horlicks, Ovaltine, Bournvita, cocoa and chocolate.

Diet for Treatment of Obesity

(Carbohydrate 80 g, protein 50 g, fat 24 g = 750 Kcalories.)

Early morning

Glass of water.

Breakfast

Half a grapefruit or 1 orange.

or

A glass of fresh or tinned diluted unsweetened fruit juice.
1 thin slice of bread (30 g), toasted if liked.
Butter and milk from daily allowance.
Tea or coffee. *No sugar or marmalade.*

Mid-morning

Glass of water, Marmite, Oxo or Bovril, or tea or coffee with milk from daily allowance.

Lunch

Clear soup or Bovril, if liked.
Medium serving meat or fish, or chicken or rabbit or egg—*not fried.*

No pastry or thick gravy or sauce.
Large serving green vegetables or salad, *or* smaller serving root vegetables.
Fruit, raw or stewed without sugar.
Tea or coffee with milk from daily allowance.

Tea
1 thin slice of bread (30 g).
Butter from daily allowance.
Marmite, tomato, lettuce or cress. *No jam.*
Tea with milk from daily allowance.

Supper
Clear soup or Bovril, if liked.
Medium serving meat or fish, or chicken or rabbit or egg—*not fried.*
No pastry or thick gravy or sauce.
Large serving green vegetables or salad.
or
Smaller serving root vegetables.
Fruit, raw or stewed without sugar.
Tea or coffee with milk from daily allowance.

Daily
Milk, 200 ml.
Butter or margarine, 7 g.
(This allows thin scrape on two slices bread.)
Saccharine may be used to sweeten.
No sugar.

The Following Foods are Suitable

White fish—*not fried.*
Very lean meat.
Chicken, rabbit or tripe.
Cod's roe—*in season*
Sweetbread.

Cheese—small portion daily.
Egg.
Fresh whole milk and butter—*in moderation.*
Wholemeal bread—*in moderation.*

Tomatoes.
Lettuce.
Watercress, mustard and cress.
Cabbage.
Cauliflower.
Spinach.
Broccoli.
French beans.
Cucumber.

Carrots and parsnips—small serving.
Asparagus.
Brussel sprouts.
Leeks.
Marrow.
Mushrooms.
Radishes.
Seakale.
Turnip—small serving.

Orange.

Grapefruit.

Apple—small, raw.

Apple—stewed without sugar.

Rhubarb.

Blackberries.

Gooseberries.

Apricots—fresh, not dried.

Lemon juice—sweetened with saccharine.

Melon.

Peach, small fresh.

Pear—small, stewed without sugar.

Plums—stewed without sugar.

Clear bone broth.

Marmite, Oxo or Bovril.

Tea, coffee.

Wheat germ—Bemax.

The Following Foods are Unsuitable and should be Avoided

Bread in excess, white flour, rice, macaroni etc.

Cakes, pastries, puddings and sweet biscuits.

Sugar.

Fat meat or fish: bacon, pork, ham, sardines, pilchards, herrings and sausages.

Thick soups, sauces and gravies.

Jam, honey, marmalade, syrup.

Tinned fruit in syrup.

All fried food.

Ice cream, olive oil, cream, mayonnaise.

Beetroot, peas, haricot beans.

Potato.

Bananas, nuts.

Sweet wines, spirits, beer, stout, sweetened drinks.

Sweets, chocolate and cocoa.

Dried fruit: dates, sultanas and prunes.

APPROXIMATE EQUIVALENT DOSES, APOTHECARIES AND METRIC SYSTEMS

Weights

Apothecary or Troy		*Metric*	*Apothecary or Troy*		*Metric*
1 oz	=	30 g	$1\frac{1}{2}$ gr		0.1 gm
4 dr	=	15 g			(or 100 mg)
$2\frac{1}{2}$ dr	=	10 g	1 gr	=	65 mg
2 dr	=	8 g	$\frac{3}{4}$ gr	=	50 mg
75 gr	=	5 g	$\frac{2}{3}$ gr	=	45 mg
1 dr	=	4 g	$\frac{1}{2}$ gr	=	32 mg
45 gr	=	3 g	$\frac{3}{8}$ gr	=	24 mg
30 gr	=	2 g	$\frac{1}{3}$ gr	=	22 mg
15 gr	=	1 g	$\frac{1}{4}$ gr	=	16 mg
10 gr	=	0.65 g	$\frac{1}{5}$ gr	=	13 mg
		(or 650 mg)	$\frac{1}{6}$ gr	=	11 mg
$7\frac{1}{2}$ gr	=	0.5 g	$\frac{1}{8}$ gr	=	8 mg
		(or 500 mg)	$\frac{1}{10}$ gr	=	6.5 mg
7 gr	=	0.45 g	$\frac{1}{12}$ gr	=	5.4 mg
		(or 450 mg)	$\frac{1}{16}$ gr	=	4 mg
6 gr	=	0.4 g	$\frac{1}{20}$ gr	=	3.2 mg
		(or 400 mg)	$\frac{1}{32}$ gr	=	2 mg
5 gr	=	0.32 g	$\frac{1}{64}$ gr	=	1 mg
		(or 320 mg)	$\frac{1}{100}$ gr	=	0.65 mg
4 gr	=	0.25 g	$\frac{1}{120}$ gr	=	0.54 mg
		(or 250 mg)	$\frac{1}{160}$ gr	=	0.4 mg
3 gr	=	0.2 g	$\frac{1}{200}$ gr	=	0.32 mg
		(or 200 mg)	$\frac{1}{250}$ gr	=	0.26 mg
$2\frac{1}{2}$ gr	=	0.16 g	$\frac{1}{320}$ gr	=	0.2 mg
		(or 160 mg)	$\frac{1}{640}$ gr	=	0.1 mg
2 gr	=	0.13 g			
		(or 130 mg)			

Liquid Measures

Apothecary		*Metric*	*Apothecary*		*Metric*
1 pint	=	568 ml	50 minims	=	3 ml
(20 fl oz)			45 minims	=	2.7 ml
12 fl oz	=	340 ml	30 minims	=	1.8 ml
8 fl oz	=	227 ml	20 minims	=	1.2 ml
6 fl oz	=	170 ml	15 minims	=	0.9 ml
4 fl oz	=	114 ml	10 minims	=	0.6 ml

3 fl oz	=	85 ml	8 minims	=	0.5 ml
2 fl oz	=	57 ml	5 minims	=	0.3 ml
1 fl oz	=	28.4 ml	3 minims	=	0.18 ml
4 fl dr	=	14 ml	2 minims	=	0.12 ml
2 fl dr	=	7 ml	1 minim	=	0.06 ml
1 fl dr	=	3.5 ml			

Weights

Apothecary		*Metric*	
60 gr	= 1 dr (ʒ)	1000 mg	= 1 gram (g)
8 dr	= 1 oz (℥)	1000 g	= 1 kilogram (kg)

Liquid Measures

Apothecary		*Metric*	
60 minims (m)	= 1 fl dr (ʒ)	1 ml	= 1000 cu mm
8 fl dr	= 1 fl oz (℥)	1000 ml	= 1 litre
20 fl oz	= 1 pint		

Household Measures

1 teaspoon	= 1 fl dr (ʒ)	= 3.5 ml
1 dessertspoon	= 2 fl dr	= 7 ml
1 tablespoon	= $\frac{1}{2}$ fl oz (℥ss)	= 14 ml

Physiological Normals

Haemoglobin (Hb)	Men:	13.5–18.0 g per dl
	Women:	11.5–16.0 g per dl
Red cells		4.0–6.0 $\times 10^{12}$/litre
White cells		4–11 $\times 10^{9}$/litre
Neutrophils		2.5–7.5 $\times 10^{9}$/litre
Lymphocytes		1.5–2.7 $\times 10^{9}$/litre
Monocytes		0.3–0.8 $\times 10^{9}$/litre
Eosinophils		0.15–0.4 $\times 10^{9}$/litre
Basophils		0–0.1 $\times 10^{9}$/litre
Fasting blood glucose		3.3–5.0 mmol/litre
Blood urea		1.7–7.0 mmol/litre
Erythrocyte sedimentation rate (ESR)		1–10 mm in 1 hour
Cerebrospinal Fluid (CSF)		
Pressure		60–160 mm of water
Protein		0.15–0.45 g/litre
Glucose		2.5–5.6 mmol/litre

CONVERSION SCALES FOR SI UNITS WITH NORMAL RANGES

(SI Units are given on the left of each scale.)

	SI units (left of scale)	Scale values	Other units (right of scale)	Scale values	Normal range
UREA	mmol/l	0, 10, 20, 30, 40, 50	mg/100ml	0, 50, 100, 150, 200, 250, 300	2.5-7.1 mmol/l
GLUCOSE	mmol/l	0, 2, 4, 6, 8, 10, 12, 14, 16, 18	mg/100ml	0, 50, 100, 150, 200, 250, 300	Fasting: 3.3-5.5 mmol/l
CALCIUM	mmol/l	0, 1, 2, 3	mg/100ml	0, 2, 4, 6, 8, 10, 12, 14	2.10-2.60 mmol/l
PHOSPHATE	mmol/l	0, 0.5, 1, 1.5, 2, 2.5, 3	mg/100ml	0, 2, 4, 6, 8, 10	0.80-1.5 mmol/l
BILIRUBIN	µmol/l	0, 20, 40, 60, 80, 100, 120, 140, 160	mg/100ml	0, 1, 2, 3, 4, 5, 6, 7, 8, 9, 10	Less than 17 µmol/l
CHOLESTEROL	mmol/l	4, 6, 8, 10, 12	mg/100ml	100, 200, 300, 400, 500	0-29 yrs: 3.10-6.20 mmol/l 30-39 yrs: 3.60-7.00 mmol/l 40-49 yrs: 3.90-8.00 mmol/l 50-59 yrs: 4.10-8.50 mmol/l
CREATININE	µmol/l	0, 200, 400, 600, 800	mg/100ml	0, 2, 4, 6, 8, 10	50-130 µmol/l
PROTEINS	g/l	10, 20, 30, 40, 50, 60, 70, 80, 90, 100	g/100ml	1, 2, 3, 4, 5, 6, 7, 8, 9, 10	Total 59-75 g/l Alb 30-45 g/l Glob: 20-38 g/l
URATE	mmol/l	0, 0.1, 0.2, 0.3, 0.4, 0.5, 0.6, 0.7, 0.8, 0.9	mg/100ml	0, 2, 4, 6, 8, 10, 12, 14	Male: 0.20-0.43 nmol/l Female: 0.14-0.33 nmol/l

Index

Abdominal pain, 78
Achalasia of the cardia, 81
Achlorhydria, 82
Acholuric jaundice, 35
Acid-fast bacilli, 71
Acromegaly, 122
ACTH, 117, 121, 175
Acyanotic congenital heart disease, 18
Addisonian crisis, 122
Addison's anaemia, 33
  disease, 121
Adrenal glands, 121
Adrenaline, 63
Adrenocorticotropic hormone, *see* ACTH
Agranulocytosis, 35, 119, 224
Allergy, 60, 224
Aminophylline, 62
Amoebic dysentery, 208
Anaemia, 30–6
  Addison's, 33
  aplastic, 35
  haemolytic, 35
  haemorrhagic, 31
  iron deficiency, 31
  macrocytic, 32, 34
  microcytic, 32
  pernicious, 33
  vitamin B_{12} deficiency, 33–5
Anaphylactoid purpura, 40
Aneurysm, 25, 167
Angina pectoris, 20
Ankylosing spondylitis, 136
Antacids, 88
Anticoagulant therapy, 23
Antihistamines, 46
Antispasmodics, 88
Aortic regurgitation, 5
Aortic stenosis, 5
Aphasia, 166
Apoplexy, 160
APT, 190
Argyll-Robertson pupils, 156
Artane, 152
Arteriogram, 154
Arthritis, rheumatoid, 131–4
  osteo, 134
Ascaris lumbricoides, 222
Ascites, 7, 97, 98
Asthma, bronchial, 44, 60
  cardiac, 6, 25, 44
Atheroma, 20, 21, 160
Atrial fibrillation, 3, 17
Atrial flutter, 4
Atrial septal defect, 18

Bacillary dysentery, 206–8
Bacterial endocarditis, 18
Barrier nursing, 187
BCG vaccination, 72
Benzyl benzoate, 178
Bereavement, 77
Blalock's operation, 18
Bradycardia, 2
Brain scan, 155
Brompton mixture, 51
Bronchial asthma, 44, 60
Bronchial carcinoma, 43, 64
Bronchiectasis, 43, 56–60
Bronchitis, acute, 49
  chronic, 50
Broncho-pneumonia, 51, 55

Carbenoxolone, 89
Carbimazole, 119
Carcinoma:
  of bronchus, 43, 64
  of colon, 102
  of oesophagus, 81
  of stomach, 91
Cardiac asthma, 6, 25, 44
Carditis, acute, 11
Carpopedal spasm, 86
Castellani's paint, 177
Cataract, 126
Cerebral embolism, 160
Cerebral haemorrhage, 26, 160
Cerebral thrombosis, 26, 160

Cerebral tumour, 153
Charcot's joints, 156
Cheyne-Stokes respiration, 7
Chickenpox, 201
Cirrhosis of liver, 96–8
  biliary, 96
  portal, 96
Clubbing of the fingers, 17
Co-arctation of aorta, 26
Coma:
  diabetic, 124, 130
  insulin, 130
  uraemic, 110
Computerised tomography, 155
Congenital heart disease, 1, 17
Congenital pulmonary artery stenosis, 6
Congestive cardiac failure, 6
Constipation, 79
Coomb's test, 35
Cor pulmonale, 50
Coronary thrombosis, 21, 44
Coryza, 45
Cough, 42
Cretinism, 120
Croup, 48
Curschmann's spirals, 44
Cushing's syndrome, 26, 121
Cyanocobalamin, 34
Cyanosis, 1, 7, 17
Cysticercosis, 222
Cystitis, 111

Diabetes insipidus, 123
Diabetes mellitus, 123–30
Diabetic coma, 124
Diarrhoea, 80
Dick test, 195
Diets, 227–232
  gastric, 88
  high fibre, 227
  in diabetes, 126
  in nephritis, 110
  in peptic ulcer, 88
Digitalis, 8
Diphtheria, 188–93
Diuretics, 9
Diverticular disease, 103
Ductus arteriosus, 18
Duodenal ulcer, 84–90
Dysentery, amoebic, 208
  bacillary, 206
Dysphagia, 33, 81
Dyspnoea, 6
Dysuria, 112

Eczema, 173
Embolism, 17, 19
Embolus, 17
Emetine, 209
Empyema thoracis, 55
Encephalitis, 205
Encephalogram, 154
Encephalopathy, 186
Endocarditis, 17
Endoscopy, 85
Enteric fever, 196–200
Epilepsy, 168–70
Ergotamine tartrate, 172
Erythema marginatum, 11
Erythema nodosum, 70
Erythrocyte sedimentation rate, 11
Exophthalmos, 118
Extra systole, 3

Fallot's tetralogy, 18
Ferrous gluconate, 33
Ferrous sulphate, 33, 99
Folic acid, 35, 99
Fouchet's test, 93
Frusemide, 9

Gamma globulin, 204
Gangrene, diabetic, 125
Gastric ulcer, 84–90
Gastric washings, 73
Gastritis, 83
Gastroscopy, 85
General paralysis of the insane (GPI), 157
Genital herpes, 217
Gigantism, 122
Glandular fever, 206
Glucose tolerance test, 124
Gluten enteropathy, 35, 98
Gold, 134, 174
Gonorrhoea, 214
Gout, 137
Grand Mal, 168
Griseofulvin, 176

Haemarthrosis, 40
Haematemesis, 85, 90, 98
Haematuria, 107
Haemodialysis, 111

Haemolysis, 34
Haemolytic anaemia, 35
Haemolytic jaundice, 93
Haemolytic streptococcus:
  in nephritis, 107
  in rheumatic fever, 10
  in scarlet fever, 195
Haemoptysis, 16, 44, 69, 73
Haemorrhagic diseases, 38
  haemophilia, 39
  of the newborn, 39
  prothrombin deficiency, 39
  purpura, 38
  thrombocytopenia, 38
Hay fever, 46
Heart, diseases of:
  acute carditis, 11, 191
  angina pectoris, 20
  bacterial endocarditis, 18
  chronic rheumatic heart disease, 16
  congenital heart disease, 17
  coronary artery disease, 20
  mitral stenosis, 16
  syphilitic aortitis, 24
Heart failure, 4
  left ventricular, 5
  right ventricular, 6
Hemiplegia, 161
Hepatic jaundice, 94
Hepatitis, 94
Hepatitis B antigen, 94
Hiatus hernia, 44, 82–3
Hodgkin's disease, 40
Hydatid cyst, 222
Hyperkalaemia, 106
Hypertension, 25–7
  benign, 26
  malignant, 26
  portal, 96, 98
Hypotensive drugs, 27
Hypothyroidism, 120
Hysteria, 170–2

Idiopathic thrombocytopenia, 39
Immunity, 67, 184
Impetigo contagiosa, 175
Infarct, 22
  myocardial, 22
Infectious hepatitis, 94–6
Influenza, 46
Insulin, 126
  coma, 129
Intal, 64
Intensive care, 75
Iron-deficiency anaemia, 31
Isoniazid, 71, 174
Isoprenaline, 62

Jacksonian epilepsy, 169
Jaundice, 92
  acholuric, 35
  haemolytic, 93
  hepatic, 94
  obstructive, 93

Kernig's sign, 146
Koilonychia, 33
Koplik's spots, 202

Laryngitis:
  acute, 48
  chronic, 48
Legionnaires' disease, 56
Leukaemia:
  acute, 36
  chronic lymphatic, 37
  chronic myeloid, 37
Lice, 178
Lobectomy, 59, 66
Lower motor neurone, 140, 142
Lumbago, 138
Lymphogranuloma inguinale, 218

Macrocytic anaemias, 34
Mantoux test, 68, 187
Mastitis, 205
Measles, 202–4
  German, 204
Melaena, 86, 90
Meningitis, 145–7
  acute lymphocytic, 147
  acute pyogenic, 145–7
  meningococcal, 145, 146
  pneumococcal, 146
  tuberculous, 147–9
Migraine, 172
Mitral stenosis, 16–7
Mitral valvotomy, 17
Multiple sclerosis, 149–51
Mumps, 204
Myxoedema, 120

Nephritis, 106–8
  acute, 107–8
  and hypertension, 26

Nephrotic syndrome, 108–9
Neurosyphilis, 155–7
Neurosis, 210
Nitrites, 21
Norethandrolone, 106

Obstructive jaundice, 93
Occult blood, 85
Oedema, 6, 9
  in heart failure, 6, 9
  in nephritis, 107, 108, 110
Oesophageal carcinoma, 81
Oliguria, 106
Oophoritis, 205
Orchitis, 205
Orthopnoea, 6
Osler's nodes, 19

Papilloedema, 26, 154
Paralysis agitans, 151
Parkinsonism, 151–2
Paroxysmal tachycardia, 4
Paul-Bunnell test, 206
Pediculosis, 178, 179
Peptic ulcer, 84–90
Perennial rhinitis, 46
Peripheral neuritis, 126
Pernicious anaemia, 33
Pertussis, 193–4
Petit mal, 169
Phaeochromocytoma, 26
Photophobia, 146, 148
Pleurisy, 44, 70
Plummer–Vinson syndrome, 33, 82
Pneumonectomy, 66
Pneumonia, 51
  broncho, 51, 55
  lobar, 51, 52
Poliomyelitis, 149
Polyarteritis nodosa, 136
Polycythaemia, 1
Polyuria, 124
Portal cirrhosis, 96
  hypertension, 96
Postural drainage, 58
Primary tuberculosis, 67
Prophylactic inoculations for children, 186
Prothrombin deficiency, 39
Pruritus, 124
Psychosis, 210
Pulmonary stenosis, 18
Pulse, 2
  bradycardia, 2
  deficit, 3, 8
  rate, 2, 8
  rhythm, 2
  tachycardia, 2
Pulsus alternans, 4, 7
Pulsus bigeminus, 4
Purpura, 36, 38, 39, 40
  anaphylactoid, 40
  Henoch's, 40
  Schönlein's, 40
  thrombocytopenic, 38
Pyelitis, 111
Pyelo-nephritis, 111
Pyloric stenosis, 86

Reiter's syndrome, 217
Renal failure:
  acute, 107–9
  chronic, 109–11
Renal transplant, 111
Respiration:
  Cheyne-Stokes, 7
  in asthma, 45, 62
  in diabetic coma, 45
  in lobar pneumonia, 45
  in uraemia, 45
Respiratory failure, 74
Rheumatic chorea, 13
Rheumatic fever, 10
Rheumatic heart disease, 11, 16
Rheumatoid arthritis, 131–4
  drugs used in, 133–4
Rhinitis, 46
Ringworm, 176
Rubella, 204

Salbutamol, 62
Scabies, 177
Scarlet fever, 195–6
Schick test, 187, 189
Schilling test, 34
Schönlein's purpura, 40
Sciatica, 138
Simmond's disease, 122
Sino-atrial node, 2, 3
Sinus arrhythmia, 3
Sinusitis, acute, 46
Skin diseases, management of, 180–3
Soft sore, 218
Spider naevi, 97

Spironolactone, 98
Sprue, 34, 98
Sputum:
  in bronchial asthma, 44
  in bronchial carcinoma, 43
  in bronchiectasis, 43
  in cardiac asthma, 44
  in lobar pneumonia, 44
  in pulmonary tuberculosis, 44
Streptococci, haemolytic, 10, 107, 195
Streptococcus viridans, 18
Streptomycin, 71, 174
Strokes, 160
St. Vitus' dance, 13
Subacute bacterial endocarditis, 17, 18
Subacute combined degeneration of the cord, 34, 152
Subarachnoid haemorrhage, 166, 167
Subdural haemorrhage, 167
Sulfasalazine, 101
Sydenham's chorea, 13
Syphilis, 215–7
  aortitis in, 24
Systemic lupus erythematosus, 135

TAB, 200
Tabes dorsalis, 155
Taenia saginata, 221
Taenia solium, 221
Tape worm, 221
Tetanus, 157–60
Tetany, 86
Thalassaemia, 35
Thrombocytopenia, 38
Thyrotoxicosis, 117–20
Tinea capitis, 176
Tinea cruris, 176
Tinea pedis, 177
Tomography, 70
Toxocariasis, 223
Tracheitis, 46
Trichinosis, 223
Trinitrin, 21
Triple vaccine, 186
Trousseau's sign, 86
Tuberculosis, 66–74
  post-primary, 68
  primary, 67
Tuberculous meningitis, 147–149
Typhoid fever, 196–200
Typhoid state, 197

Ulcerative colitis, 99–102
Upper motor neurone, 140, 142
Uraemia, 109
Urinary tract infections, 111
Urine concentration test, 109

Varicella, 201
Venereal disease, 214–20
Ventricular septal defect, 18
Ventriculography, 154
Vitamins, 113–6
  Vitamin A, 113
  Vitamin B, 114
  Vitamin B_{12}, 34
  Vitamin C, 114
  Vitamin D, 114
  Vitamin K, 115–6
Vomiting, 80
  cerebral, 80
  psychological, 80

Whitfield's ointment, 176, 177
Whooping cough, 43, 193
Widal test, 197